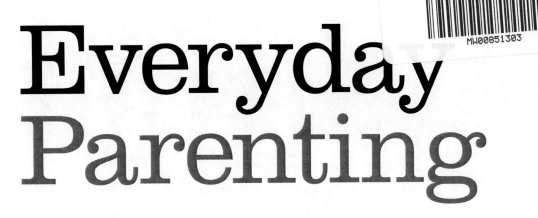

Everyday Parenting

A Professional's Guide to Building Family Management Skills

Thomas J. Dishion

Elizabeth A. Stormshak

Kathryn A. Kavanagh

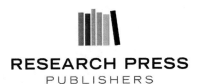

RESEARCH PRESS
PUBLISHERS

2612 North Mattis Avenue ● Champaign, Illinois 61822 ● [800] 519-2707 ● www.researchpress.com

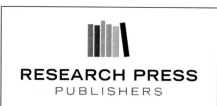

RESEARCH PRESS
PUBLISHERS

Copies of this book may be ordered from Research Press at the address given
on the title page.

Composition by Jeff Helgesen
Cover design by Linda Brown, Positive I.D. Graphic Design, Inc.
Printed by Seaway Printing Co.

ISBN: 978–0-87822-658-0
Library of Congress Control Number 2011931020

To my children, with whom I continue the journey of family life,
and to the friends and colleagues who have supported the development
of this family intervention, often with too little pay and a great deal
of employment uncertainty.

—Tom Dishion

To my family, who has supported me throughout my career; to my mentor,
Karen Bierman, who provided me with a foundation of learning
and support at Penn State; and to my colleagues at the University of Oregon,
who are great people to work and laugh with.

—Beth Stormshak

To all the families who have shared their wisdom and their struggles. Through
your engagement in these materials and activities, you have helped us create
useful, commonsense parenting support for the next generation of families.

—Kate Kavanagh

Contents

Figures   *vii*

Handouts   *ix*

Preface   *xiii*

Acknowledgments   *xv*

Overview: Everyday Parenting Curriculum   1

Sessions

1   Positive Behavior Support: Parent Requests and Child Cooperation   17

2   Positive Behavior Support: Parent Praise for Positive Behavior   29

3   Behavior-Change Plans: Instruction and Incentives   41

4   Behavior-Change Plans: Reviewing, Revising, and Reducing Barriers to Change   59

5   Monitoring Daily Activities: Daily Structure and Listening   71

6   SANE Guidelines for Limit Setting: Identifying Consequences and Monitoring Questions   85

7   Proactive Limit-Setting Plan: Giving Consequences and Ignoring Mild Problem Behavior   103

8   Limit-Setting Challenges and Emotion Regulation   121

9   Improving Family Relationships with Negotiation   133

10   Choosing Solutions to Family Problems   147

11   Proactive Parenting and Planning: Positive Routines That Reduce Stress   157

12   Shared Family Routines: Communication Skills That Promote Engagement and Enjoyment   171

Appendix: Child and Family Feedback Form   187

References   189

About the Authors   193

Figures

Figure 1   Conceptual framework for the Everyday Parenting curriculum and the Family Check-Up (FCU).   3

Figure 2   The Family Check-Up in context.   6

Figure 3   Developmental changes in parenting practices relevant to child contexts.   7

Figure 4   The cyclical behavior-change process.   9

Figure 5   Family management in relation to other factors.   15

Figure 6   Parenting change process: The COACH model.   16

Figure 7   *Top:* How coercion works to disrupt family interactions. *Bottom:* How a successful intervention can support family management.   18

Figure 8   The ABCs of positive family change.   30

Figure 9   Parental limit setting and positive behavior support in the path of life.   87

Figure 10   A parent's role in developing good communication and a positive parent–child relationship.   173

Handouts

The CD that accompanies this book contains pdf files of all handouts used in this program.

1A: Pinpointing Positive Behaviors   25

1B: Making Positive Requests   26

1C: Session 1 Tracking Form (Completed Example)   27

1D: Session 1 Tracking Form   28

2A: Giving Praise   37

2B: Session 2 Tracking Form (Completed Example)   38

2C: Session 2 Tracking Form   39

3A: Ideas for Incentives   51

3B: Alternative Incentives   52

3C: Behavior Plan for Older Children (Completed Example)   53

3D: Behavior Plan for Younger Children (Completed Example)   54

3E: Setting Up a Plan with Your Child   55

3F: Behavior Plan for Older Children   56

3G: Behavior Plan for Younger Children   57

3H: Questions to Ask When Creating an Incentive Plan   58

4A: What If? Behavior Plan Scenarios   67

4B: Parent in the Mirror: Beliefs About Change   68

4C: Self-Statements Log   69

5A: The Four Cs of Monitoring   79

5B: Networking Example   80

5C: Parent Self-Assessment for Limit Setting   81

5D: Active Listening Check-Up   83

5E: Setting Limits: Parent Assessment   84

6A: House Rules   95

6B: SANE Limit-Setting Guidelines   96

6C: Setting Limits Activity   97

6D: Questions That May Lead to Useful Information   98

6E: Home Practice: Questioning   99

6F: Tracking Rules   100

6G: Getting Useful Information from Your Child   101

7A: Types of Consequences   113

7B: Setting the Rules, Setting the Consequences   114

7C: Four Guidelines for Giving Consequences   115

7D: Time-Out Sequence   116

7E: Examples of When to Ignore   117

7F: Steps for Using Time-Out   118

7G: Changing Habits and Behaviors   119

8A: Warning Signs for Problem Behavior   128

8B: Rules and Consequences for Serious Problem Behavior   129

8C: CALM Guidelines   130

8D: Challenges to Time-Out   131

9A: Negotiation Questionnaire   141

9B: Negotiation Don'ts   142

9C: What, When, and Where of Negotiation   143

9D: Examples of Neutral Problem Statements for School-Age Children   144

9E: Bringing Up a Problem: Checklist   145

10A: Family Negotiation Form (Completed Example)   155

10B: Family Negotiation Form   156

11A: Deciding When to Use What   166

11B: PLAN for Proactive Parenting   167

11C: Proactive Structuring Checklist   168

11D: Gathering Information   169

12A: Family Communication Profile   182

12B: Shared Family Routine Form (Completed Example)   183

12C: Shared Family Routine Form   184

12D: Communication (Handout for Your Child)   185

Preface

The Everyday Parenting model is an adaptation of the social learning approach to parent training, family therapy, and couples therapy (Patterson, 1973; Patterson, Reid, Jones, & Conger, 1975). The authors of this book were trained in intervention protocols that were originally developed at the Oregon Social Learning Center (OSLC), where Jerry Patterson founded and led a unique program of innovation and science dedicated to helping families with aggressive children (see Patterson, 1982, for a summary). The social learning treatment model, later known as the *social interactional model* (Patterson & Reid, 1984; Patterson, Reid, & Dishion, 1992), was heavily predicated on behavior analysis, with greater emphasis placed on changing functional dynamics and less emphasis placed on cognitive aspects contributing to family interaction and aggression. There was no doubt that the treatment worked, because each case was evaluated by observers who visited treatment families' homes before, during, and after therapy, and the families' "total aversive behavior" (TAB) scores were graphed for all the center to see (Reid, 1978). There was no place to hide if you were a therapist and your family was not responding well to treatment!

Case conferences were focused on families whose TAB scores were not changing, and the group mobilized into creative problem solving. These discussions generated new constructs, such as "monitoring," "family stress," and "peer deviance," that were later plugged into research and became the target of future interventions. With intense effort, mutual support, and considerable laughter, the work continued. The OSLC model that emerged from this process became central to treating children's and adolescents' conduct problems with a family-centered approach (Forgatch & Patterson, 2010), to supporting foster and biological parents in multidimensional treatment foster care (Smith & Chamberlain, 2010), and to supporting parents of children in elementary school (Eddy, Reid, Stoolmiller, & Fetrow, 2003). In many ways, all members of the research team contributed to each new direction the intervention model would take.

The OSLC model was also applied to the prevention of alcohol and drug use and abuse in adolescence (Dishion, Reid, & Patterson, 1988). From this development sprang the initial version of the Everyday Parenting intervention—the Adolescent Transitions Program (Dishion, Andrews, Kavanagh, & Soberman, 1996; Dishion & Kavanagh, 2003). Through this program, researchers at the Child and Family Center used systematic intervention outcome research to develop a front-end motivational intervention called the Family Check-Up (Dishion & Kavanagh, 2003; Dishion, Kavanagh, & Dionne, 1998). In the process, an early focus on developing self-regulation in the context of adolescent peer groups was dropped because of iatrogenic effects that resulted from peer contagion (Dishion & Andrews, 1995; Dishion, McCord, & Poulin, 1999). Throughout the course of 24 years of amending and refining the intervention, the Everyday Parenting approach evolved to its present form.

The model benefited from other family-centered work in the field as well, including group interventions with parents that are coordinated with those in preschool settings (Webster-Stratton & Reid, 2010), interventions that target children with problem behavior (Zisser & Eyberg, 2010), those that target youth with conduct problems (Kazdin, 2010), and those that target adolescents (Henggeler & Schaeffer, 2010; Liddle, 2010; Waldron & Brody, 2010).

The Everyday Parenting model has recently been applied to prevention and treatment with families of young children (Shaw, Dishion, Supplee, Gardner, & Arnds, 2006; Dishion et al., 2008). It has been found to be as appropriate for use with families with young children as it is for families with adolescents; however, specific parenting constructs, such as parental monitoring, change in definition and emphasis with children's development (see Dishion & McMahon, 1999).

The Everyday Parenting intervention model is "social interactional" in that it prioritizes targeting and changing family interactions that occur frequently and that are functionally related to the family's behavioral health. The term *everyday* underscores the importance of addressing habitual interaction patterns that are difficult to change because of their repetitive nature. These patterns may also be heavily influenced by circumstances such as lack of resources, ethnic culture, parent depression, or divorce and remarriage (e.g., Conger et al., 2002; Elder, Caspi, & Van Nguyen, 1986; Forgatch, Patterson, & Skinner, 1988; Hetherington, 1988; Shaw, Gilliom, Ingoldsby, & Nagin, 2003). To effectively support parents and other caregivers, daily parenting practices must be linked with the realities of the family's situation. When the skills for that purpose are provided, child and adult mental health is reinforced and maintained.

Acknowledgments

We acknowledge the hard work, compassion, and perseverance of the therapists who have worked with families on our various intervention projects for many years and have contributed to the intervention model described in this book. In particular, we recognize Michel Markstrom, Nancy Weisel, Trina McCartney, Annette Ramsey, Genie Gomez, Denise Lopez-Haugen, Mary Omerife, Kevin Moore, Becky Higgens, and Alison Prescott.

We express our gratitude to Anne Gill and Michel Markstrom for their careful reading of previous versions of this curriculum and the valuable feedback they provided. Daniel Shaw, Melvin Wilson, and Anne Gill are gratefully acknowledged for their collegial support and collaboration on the Early Steps project and for helping broaden the focus of the Everyday Parenting curriculum to include young childhood through adolescence.

Several individuals have worked directly and indirectly on previous versions of this curriculum. We appreciate the contributions of Larry Soberman and David Andrews to the original Parent Focus curriculum, which formed the basis of the Everyday Parenting curriculum. In the early 1990s, colleagues at Oregon Research Institute tested the Parent Focus curriculum in rural Oregon communities. This work clarified the need for another round of revisions. We specifically acknowledge Tony Biglan, Carol Metzler, and Blair Irvine for their collaborations and insightful suggestions about how best to revise the curriculum. In addition, Peggy Veltman is appreciated for her contributions to the curriculum and her research on implementing the program in several middle schools in Eugene, Oregon.

This work would not have been possible without the continuous support since 1987 from the National Institute on Drug Abuse (grants DA 07031, DA 018374, DA 13773) and more recent support for the application of the intervention model to early childhood (grant DA 016110). We are privileged to conduct our work in a nation with a well-organized system for funding and supporting science that directly improves the lives of children and families.

Everyday Parenting Curriculum

OVERVIEW OF THE CURRICULUM

The Everyday Parenting curriculum can be used while guiding individual family therapy, while leading parent groups, and while training therapists, counselors, social workers, and other professionals to work collaboratively with parents of children and adolescents in clinical, school, and community-based mental health settings. The skills emphasized emerged from longitudinal research on the origins of child and of adolescent problem behavior and from the extensive parenting intervention literature. The Everyday Parenting curriculum has been used with parents in urban and rural settings across the United States for more than 20 years and with parents of adolescents in Spain and in Quebec, Canada (translated into Spanish and French, respectively). In addition, the curriculum has met the needs of families across a wide range of cultural groups. Evaluations of the effectiveness of the Everyday Parenting program, the EcoFIT model, and related parent interventions at OSLC with thousands of families are readily available (see Dishion & Kavanagh, 2003; Dishion & Stormshak, 2007; Snyder, Reid, & Patterson, 2003).

The data have shown that the parenting skills and communication processes taught in the program reduce negative parent–child interactions and decrease youth problem behavior at home and at school. Several other reports summarize research concerning successful implementation of this program within the school environment. Moreover, simply providing feedback to parents about their parenting patterns, in the form of the Family Check-Up (FCU), leads to long-term changes in child and adolescent problem behavior that have been mediated by changes in parenting practices. The key to working with this curriculum in any setting is to approach the material with a collaborative mind-set and respect for cultural differences in family management and parenting styles.

Note

Although this book is written for use by counselors, social workers, and other mental health professionals, the term *therapist* is used to denote the specialist who is leading the sessions.

The content of the 12 parent sessions is divided into three broad areas of parenting skills. As shown in Figure 1, monitoring and proactive parenting are the common features of all three domains targeted in the Everyday Parenting curriculum. Monitoring refers to parents' overall involvement with their children and direct and indirect knowledge of their children's safety, behavior, feelings, experiences, and whereabouts (for more detail, see Dishion & McMahon, 1999). Proactive parenting focuses on planning and using skillful strategies to overcome parenting obstacles—for example, planning a day's activities for a young child that takes into account transition times, stimulation levels, and feelings and emotions. Similarly, for adolescents, planning to help an adolescent structure his or her day realistically will provide a framework for the youth to meet goals in school or other activities. Being proactive and monitoring children and adolescents form the basis of what might be called *mindful parenting*. Simply put, mindful parenting is parenting that emphasizes attention to everyday details.

Figure 1 demonstrates the best sequence in which to make comprehensive behavior change in families who commit to the full program. Nearly all behavioral approaches to family change indicate that it is best to begin with the use of incentives (contingent positive reinforcement), move to setting limits, and end with family problem solving and proactive structuring. The rationale for this sequence is twofold. First, to adequately manage child and adolescent behavior, it is important to rely on positive reinforcement (incentives) for behavior change. In fact, we hold that the ratio of positive reinforcement to correction should be roughly 4:1, in that for every time a parent sets a limit, we would hope to see four incidents of positive reinforcement. We assume that the 4:1 ratio of reinforcement to correction creates a more positive context for behavior management. Second, it is clear that skills such as problem solving and basic communication are beneficial to children and families at all ages, but parents are less likely to be successful at learning these skills if they are not proficient in the use of positive reinforcement and limit setting. Daily negative or coercive family interactions are likely to undermine the positive parent–child relationships required for problem-solving interactions.

The Everyday Parenting curriculum addresses three dimensions of parenting:

Positive behavior support is addressed in Sessions 1 through 4. Parents practice stepping away from their problematic situations and learn the usefulness of monitoring and tracking daily child and adolescent behavior to recognize and reinforce positive behavior. The foundation of positive behavior support is parents' ability to make effective requests of their children or adolescents. An effective request is clear, specific, and nonblaming. A written behavior-change plan is a tool to help parents focus their attention on and respond consistently to positive behavior. Parents practice using praise when they review the contract and give earned incentives. The goal is for children and adolescents to eventually maintain positive behaviors because of parental praise and attention. Practicing constructive and specific requests and using them consistently help ensure success.

FIGURE 1   Conceptual framework for the Everyday Parenting curriculum and the Family Check-Up (FCU).

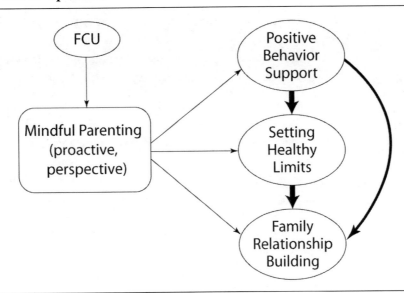

Setting healthy limits is addressed in Sessions 5 through 8. These sessions focus on specifying clear rules and expectations to children and youths, ranging from routine behaviors such as homework to serious problems such as drug use. A central component of the limit-setting sessions is the introduction of the SANE guidelines for responding to inappropriate child behaviors. SANE refers to consequences that are **S**mall, that **A**void punishing the parent, and that are **N**onabusive and **E**ffective. Parents also identify beliefs and practices that may interfere with effective limit setting. Separating negative emotions from discipline and adopting smaller consequences that can be used more consistently and more often are critical components of the limit-setting skills parents learn.

Parental monitoring is essential for healthy limit setting, which emphasizes rules and offers methods for tracking youths' out-of-home time by networking with other parents, the school, and the community. We found that parents often feel they have minimal ability to monitor behavior when their youths are outside the home. Some believe that as children get older, parents should back away and let them make their own choices about friends, drug use, and other social activities. Another common concern expressed in parent groups is that increasing supervision communicates lack of trust and interferes with an adolescent's sense of privacy. It certainly is true that less supervision is needed when there is little problem behavior and a high level of trust, and an unexplained increase in monitoring could actually have negative effects on the parent–youth relationship. When youths are involved in problem behavior, however, parental monitoring is not a matter of trust but of parents providing support, safety, and protection.

Our work, and that of many others, has consistently shown the positive effects of parental monitoring on youth outcomes and as protection against negative peer influences. This area of parenting is critical to reducing a youth's risk for drug use, precocious sexual behaviors, school expulsion, and delinquency.

Communication and problem-solving skills are a part of many of the early parent sessions and are addressed exclusively in Sessions 9 through 12. A self-assessment of parent–youth communication about adolescent topics such as boy–girl relations or alcohol and drugs sets the stage for these sessions.

Listening skills are given particular attention to help parents make the transition into a new role with their children. It is typical for parents to offer advice and solve problems when children are younger. With adolescents, it is helpful for parents to understand that they can learn more about their youths' decision making by listening carefully and observing. Although listening is a critical skill when one is parenting adolescents, listening carefully to younger children is also necessary for understanding their early decision-making skills, and it is formative in terms of their perspective, compassion, empathy, and ability to develop positive relationships with other children.

Problem-solving skills provide a structure to help families negotiate conflict in general and, in particular, to give adolescents opportunities to have a voice in the family. There are many times when it is possible to provide children with choices of activities and the like. In adolescence, it becomes developmentally appropriate for youths to want input in family decision making. When the youth is denied access to this process, an increase in parent–youth conflict will likely result. Problem-solving skills provide a structure for encouraging adolescent input in situations that caregivers deem appropriate.

The parent is the leader in the problem-solving process. At the hub of problem solving is making neutral problem statements. This skill is consistent with an effective request in that it is also nonblaming, specific, and clear. The second major skill is generating alternatives, a process during which children and parents generate ideas and withhold criticism or reactions. Selecting a course of action is the final stage, and it involves weighing the pros and cons of various choices. These skills emphasize the changing parent–child relationship and present a process for handling problem behaviors. We suggest that with some children's and youths' problems, this process can be an alternative to imposing a consequence. Teens' participation in solving minor, recurring problems, such as not cleaning up after using the bathroom or leaving food around the house, helps them develop these skills for use in situations they will encounter with friends and other adults. The sessions about family problem solving are structured and use a lot of role-plays and humor while practicing the skills, which often makes them parent favorites.

ECOFIT

The Everyday Parenting curriculum is the skill and training component of our ecological approach to family intervention and treatment (EcoFIT) (Dishion & Stormshak, 2007; Stormshak & Dishion, 2002). Several unique features of EcoFIT warrant attention with respect to the use of the Everyday Parenting curriculum. First and foremost, our strategy is to adapt and tailor interventions to meet each family's needs. Although all empirically supported intervention programs that target parenting certainly adapt interventions to family needs, in EcoFIT, we systematically use assessments to identify parenting strengths and weaknesses and collaborate with parents to identify change priorities. We propose that this strategy reduces the number of sessions needed and engages a wider range of children and families in interventions that improve parenting. Thus, as shown in Figure 2, we provide a variety of settings in which the information in the Everyday Parenting curriculum can be communicated both to caregivers, who have a range of intervention needs, and to children and adolescents across the age spectrum.

A second characteristic of the EcoFIT approach is periodic and sometimes brief interventions during times of developmental and contextual transition. For example, the early childhood years are an extended transition period during which the child's rapid development of cognitive (e.g., self-regulation), motor (e.g., walking and running), and language skills demand change in parenting strategies and family ecology. The optimal service settings in which to implement EcoFIT are those that ensure continual contact with a child and family during a specific developmental period. We have implemented the model with children whose families were enrolled in the Women, Infants, and Children (WIC) nutrition program during the children's early years and found that even a few sessions resulted in statistically reliable changes in parenting and in child behavior (Dishion et al., 2008; Shaw, Dishion, Supplee, Gardner, & Arnds, 2006). We also implemented this model in public schools to guide and support children, early adolescents, and families during transitions (Dishion & Kavanagh, 2003). Taken together, both strategies offer continuity in mental health service to families during an extended period of time. The approach is most akin to a health maintenance model of mental health service delivery and least like a medical disease model of intervention. Specifically, we propose that six to eight sessions can lead to relatively large effects for children and adolescents if they are delivered skillfully and strategically during the course of 2 to 3 years.

A third unique element of EcoFIT is that motivation to change is actively and explicitly addressed at all stages of the intervention process. The FCU provides an assessment and addresses parents' motivation to change (see Miller & Rollnick, 2002). During the course of the intervention, we address motivation at several stages of the change process. For example, during implementation of the Everyday Parenting curriculum, we provide motivation-related concerns for each skill and draw from the work of OSLC while addressing resistance to change. In addition, we provide brief motivational support for families to reinforce persistence and maintenance of change.

This ecologically sensitive intervention acknowledges the importance of considering the family's needs with respect to a variety of social and community resources. For example, in middle childhood and adolescence, it is critical to

FIGURE 2   The Family Check-Up in context.

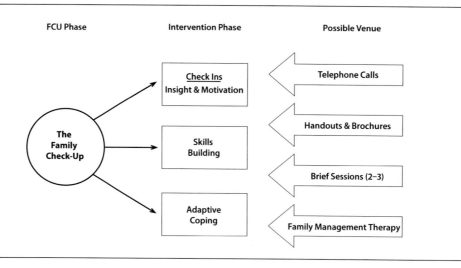

connect interventions and assessments of children and families with relevant staff members in school environments. In a child's early years, we actively link family intervention services to social services that support the health and education of young children, including preschool programs such as Early Head Start and Head Start.

Thus the Everyday Parenting curriculum and EcoFIT are relevant for families with children ages 2 through 17. Most points on this large developmental spectrum require similar sets of parenting skills. Figure 3 provides an overview of the developmental perspective on changing contexts and socialization emphases from early childhood through adolescence. During infancy, the primary emphasis of parenting involves the caregiver's responsiveness to the infant's needs. Responsiveness and warmth set the foundation for a secure and trusting parent–child relationship. Later in childhood, this relationship builds on shared activities and routines that families develop and engage in daily. Later, parents' ability to remain involved in the lives of their adolescents is critical to maintaining a positive parent–child relationship. The developmental overview provided in Figure 3 shows a hierarchical integration perspective on parental influences on children. A parent's behavior management skills are strengthened in the context of a positive parent–child relationship. Behavior management emerges in the form of key, effortful, caregiver skills that require positive behavior support (tracking, monitoring, and contingent positive reinforcement) and limit setting, beginning with toddlers and preschoolers. These behavior management skills remain instrumental throughout childhood and adolescence, but as the child becomes more involved and self-regulated in other social contexts, parents may rely more on good communication and on monitoring adolescents as the youths go about the business of living in a world independent of the family.

In middle childhood, school becomes a critical social context for children's adaptation in that it defines the child's acceptance by peers and provides the

FIGURE 3   **Developmental changes in parenting practices relevant to child contexts.**

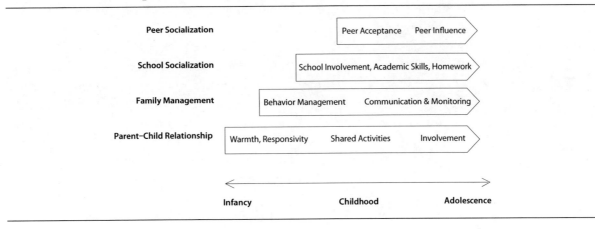

training experiences necessary for the development and refinement of academic skills (Kellam, 1990). Parental attention, awareness, and involvement in contexts such as schools are likely to be instrumental for the success of many children and adolescents with respect to their peer relationships and the development of academic skills. As children become increasingly able to self-regulate, school systems often require a great deal of self-management in terms of demands for homework completion and studying. Parents' interest, involvement, communication, and monitoring practices are vital to adolescents' development of autonomy and skilled functioning. Biologically, as children become adolescents, they are increasingly interested in establishing and maintaining friendships, some of which may be relatively independent of families. Early on, parents can have a role in setting up children for success by getting youths involved in activities that place them strategically in prosocial peer groups. In the event that youths cluster into groups based on problem behavior, then parents' monitoring skills become increasingly instrumental in reducing negative peer influence during adolescence.

Cultural sensitivity is an inherent strength of the intervention's ecological perspective. The EcoFIT model addresses both cultural and regional contexts, and it incorporates the specific needs of African American, American Indian, European American, Latino, and low-income families who live in suburban, urban, and rural communities. The intervention design incorporates the distinct aspects of the family's culture as part of the treatment approach. The Family Check-Up is the cornerstone for tailoring and adapting the intervention to the family and the point at which cultural issues can be addressed in terms of treatment goals. Therapists, for example, provide home visit sessions in Spanish to Latino families, have knowledge of the specific cultural aspects of family life and child rearing in African American and Latino homes, and are sensitive to regional, historical, and population density issues. Moreover, by building the intervention around family-identified needs and goals, cultural and personal perspectives of the family become central to the intervention.

The specific procedures for the Family Check-Up are described in detail by Dishion and Stormshak (2007). Briefly, the cornerstone of EcoFIT is the FCU, which is specifically designed for two purposes: (1) to motivate parents to change their daily parenting practices and (2) to tailor interventions to best meet the needs of families, taking into account their strengths and weaknesses in parenting, their current available resources, and their motivation to change. The FCU is modeled on the Drinker's Check-Up, following the principles of motivational interviewing developed and articulated by Miller and colleagues (Miller & Rollnick, 2002). The FCU consists of three sessions: (1) an initial contact session, (2) an assessment session that includes direct observations of family interaction, and (3) a feedback session during which the therapist reviews with the parent the assessment results and collaborates with caregivers to identify appropriate change targets in their parenting. A Child and Family Feedback form is provided in the appendix so that the therapist can combine the FCU with the Everyday Parenting curriculum, as we recommend. Therapists could design their own assessment strategies and perhaps use the feedback form to provide caregivers with an idea of their current strengths and aspects of their parenting that need attention. This collaborative process with parents is designed to enhance motivation, to use assessment to help parents engage in decision making, and to evaluate the focus and intensity of the intervention on a case-by-case basis.

THE CHANGE PROCESS

It is unrealistic to expect that behavior change will result automatically without some continued support to the clients. The habitual nature of the behavior and the emotional and ecological climate affect the pace and dynamics of behavior change. Meaningful, long-term change is often cyclical and moves from insight and motivation to skills and training to adaptation to one's life. For example, supporting parents' use of positive reinforcement is likely to begin with some sense that the child and family could benefit from contingent positive responses to the child's positive behavior, then to progress to developing skills in reinforcement, such as learning to use a point or a sticker chart, and then to integrating and adapting the principle of reinforcement to other aspects of child rearing, perhaps to other children or other behaviors. This cycle is shown in Figure 4.

The Family Check-Up sets the stage for parents' motivation to lead the change process in their families. One conclusion that may result from the FCU feedback session with a parent is that more support may be needed to enact the change. This support is most likely to come in the form of periodic (e.g., weekly) meetings with the parent and child or perhaps with parents' participation in parenting groups. The Everyday Parenting curriculum is designed to facilitate working with parents to change parenting practices. It is at this stage that the therapist becomes more actively involved in the behavior-change cycle. By and large, therapist involvement is the most intense during the skill development stage because the therapist leads the structuring of

FIGURE 4   The cyclical behavior-change process.

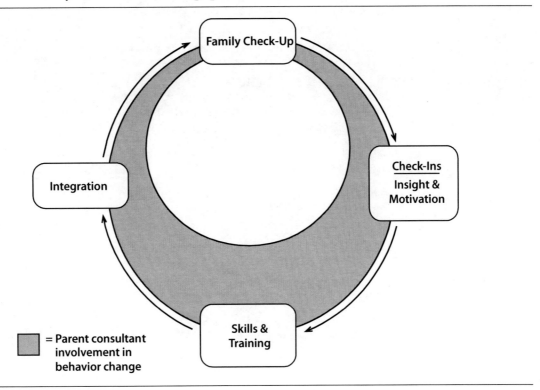

interactions that promote skill development within a family ecology. Once a family has developed the skills and is maintaining family and child behavior gains, the therapist becomes less active and often follows the parents' lead in finding solutions to difficulties and barriers.

Paradoxically, clients often resist changes they may have endorsed at the outset of an intervention plan. For example, when a therapist is encouraging skills-training interventions, it is quite common for clients to resist change in the form of avoidance of sessions, negativity about the child or the behavior-change plan, helplessness, hopelessness, or behavioral signs of distrust and premature quitting. It is the therapist's task to effectively respond to patterns of client resistance in the interest of the child's and family's health and well-being. More information about managing resistance is presented throughout this manual.

Resistance to change is addressed at the outset by using motivational interviewing procedures. A key feature of motivational interviewing is to encourage clients to choose from a flexible menu of intervention options (Miller & Rollnick, 2002). For example, if parent groups are the only means offered for learning to change parenting practices, then many parents would be resistant to change because they may be reluctant to attend a parent group or simply could not fit attendance into their schedule. The ability to choose an appropriate intervention option empowers caregivers to continue their involvement. Our menu of intervention options is based on the content provided in the

Everyday Parenting curriculum, as shown in Figure 1. In addition to directly focusing on issues of motivation, we propose a set of steps that are useful for structuring each session, which will help to counter resistance and to develop parents' successful implementation of the skills.

SIX STEPS FOR STRUCTURING SESSIONS

The first step in carrying out a successful session is to come prepared with all the necessary tools. For example, if you are going to suggest role-play examples, it's good to have those written out ahead of time. Getting off to a good start is the second step and is helped by leading off with open-ended questions, which are suggested for each session. The third step is to set an agenda that helps structure the time and offers a road map of where you would like to go during the session. This step also enables parents to contribute their ideas about what should be discussed during your meeting time. The fourth step is to focus on process and to cultivate awareness of the parents during each session by observing thoughts and feelings and then responsively structuring the content and pacing. A fifth and central step in Everyday Parenting is the use of role-plays of family management skills and interactional processes to facilitate in-session practice. This practice makes it possible to provide supportive feedback and to develop the parents' abilities and sense of self-efficacy when they use these skills at home with their children. The sixth step is to create tailored and relevant home practice "experiments" of the session content. When parents feel that you understand their situation, they are more likely to engage in the home practice and be ready to make changes in their behavior.

USING ROLE-PLAY WHILE SUPPORTING FAMILY MANAGEMENT SKILLS

Working with parents to change habitual parenting reactions is an active, effortful process. Abstract discussion of parenting principles is unlikely to lead to change for the majority of parents. Behavior-change efforts will be most effective when parents practice the parenting skills in this curriculum. Practice facilitates the performance of new skills in the everyday life of the family. To support the process of behavior change, the therapist seeks to free the parent from being a victim of habit and emotion. For example, coming home to a house that is a mess may justifiably make a parent angry, but when the parent can make an effective request rather than unleash a critical, angry tirade, all family members will benefit.

Although parents may have the best intentions, they may find it difficult to enact the skills they know are so important. Role-playing is a valuable tool for empowering parents to make positive changes in their family interactions. Results from randomized interventions, in fact, reveal that when therapists use role-play to teach and support parenting skills, the positive effects of the intervention service are increased (Kaminski, Valle, Filene, & Boyle, 2008). Role-playing with parents is considered to be the "grist of the mill" in effective parent training (Forgatch, Bullock, & Patterson, 2004).

Two critical characteristics of role-play must be remembered when using this curriculum. First, role-play is most effective for conveying parenting skills that require emotion regulation. Examples include making effective requests, stating rules, using time-out, giving consequences, listening, and making neutral problem statements during problem solving. All these behaviors share one key dynamic: Regulation of emotion is necessary while implementing skillful and tactful parenting. Using role-play to practice these parenting behaviors will increase the likelihood that the behaviors will be used in day-to-day family life.

Second, the optimal strategy for engaging parents and children in role-play is the "wrong way/right way" approach. It involves first practicing the "wrong way" to engage in an interpersonal interaction and then practicing the "right way." A particular advantage to this approach is that it is far less anxiety provoking to practice responding inappropriately and ineffectively. To begin the role-play process, it is helpful if the therapist "plays" the parent while the parent "plays" the youth. For example:

> **Therapist:** I'd like you to be Linda and act like you are ignoring me when I ask you to pick up your things.
>
> **Parent:** *Ignoring the therapist while attending to the TV.*
>
> **Therapist:** What's the matter with you, are you trying to make my life difficult? Why can't you answer me when I ask you to do something?
>
> **Parent and therapist:** *Laughing.*
>
> **Therapist:** So what did I do wrong when I was reacting to Linda's ignoring?

Wrong-way role-plays are only as useful as the debriefing that follows. Having parents articulate the negative consequences of an inappropriate parenting reaction helps them learn to discriminate productive from nonproductive exchanges. It is especially helpful to list all aspects of the "wrong way" with the parents. The next phase is to role-play the "right way" to engage in an interpersonal interaction. Each section of this curriculum describes family management skills that can be used to structure role-plays. It is especially helpful to have parents first list what they see as aspects of an effective response. Following the parents' lead, it is then helpful for the therapist to add to the list. It is especially important to limit the focus to no more than two to three skills for the parents to keep in mind while enacting the role-play.

> **Therapist:** Great! So making eye contact, staying calm, and being specific in your request would be a big improvement. In this situation what could you say that would fit those three qualities?
>
> **Parent:** Linda, please pick up your toys in the hallway now.

> **Therapist:** Great, now say that to me as I act like Linda and watch TV (*therapist sits back in chair and pretends to watch TV*).

When the parent enacts the parenting skill, it is crucial to motivate him or her by expressing support. It is a mistake to fail to support even the small enactments. Following are ENACT guidelines for therapists to help them conduct effective role-plays during sessions:

> **E** = Enough practice and corrective feedback are provided so that parents can successfully use the skill at home.
>
> **N** = Negative affect is modeled in the wrong-way role-play and then replaced with a positive parenting skill in the right-way role-play.
>
> **A** = Actively structure role-play sessions to encourage parents' participation and enjoyment.
>
> **C** = Clear directions and examples are critical to parent success.
>
> **T** = Tailor the role-play to the current skill level of the parent and then build on success by using corrective feedback and shaping.

Most of the sessions in this curriculum include examples and material that support the role-play process when working with parents on family management skills. Family change will be most pronounced and successful if all key family members participate. For example, role-plays that include only the father would be less effective than those that include both parents, regardless of whether the family is a biological family or consists of an unmarried couple cooperating on parenting, grandparent–parent dyads, or a blended family. It is often appropriate to demonstrate or role-play a skill by including the child or the child and siblings in the intervention session.

INCLUDING CHILDREN IN PARENTING SESSIONS

Children as young as 3 or 4 years can be included in discussions about incentives, rules, household changes, and so on. These discussions can become role-plays during which the parent and child enact the change while the therapist offers support and guidance.

There are many benefits to including children in sessions during which family management skills are developed and supported. For example, children know best what incentive will motivate them to learn a new behavior (e.g., coming to dinner when called) or maintain a current behavior parents desire (e.g., cleaning their room, making their bed), or what privilege they most want to maintain through good behavior (e.g., watching their favorite TV program, staying up past a set bedtime). Including children in discussions about problem areas can inform both caregivers and clinicians about the various factors at play from the child's perspective, and this information can be used to more effectively tailor the intervention. Including children in role-plays can be instructive at multiple levels and obviously is closer to reality than having a therapist or a parent play the role of the child. Involving children in practice sessions can be particularly useful when parents are ready to practice and implement a new skill that they have been working on with the therapist. Before trying it on their own at home, they can sharpen the skill with the therapist's follow-up feedback. And, significantly, role-playing with the child can facilitate parent confidence and competence.

That said, timing and context for involving children in sessions are critical to ensure success. The major contraindication for involving children is that they may be so noncompliant or collusive that role-play enactments will be unsuccessful and the parent will leave the session discouraged and feeling certain that the children's behavior is unmanageable. This scenario may apply to just one child, or it may play out when all siblings are brought into a session and they engage in collusive and undermining behaviors.

The most important aspect of including children in role-plays is to empower the parent to use the family management skill at home every day. Children's participation in sessions should be structured to improve the parent–child relationship and to empower the parent in a leadership role. Attention to the following factors will help promote this outcome:

> **E** = Elicit from parents the most likely family situation in which the targeted parenting skill will be needed.

> **M** = Model targeted behaviors for parents before children are brought into the session to ensure a successful parent enactment.

> **P** = Proactively plan for potential problems together with parents before children are brought into a role-play enactment.

> **O** = Observe and respect parents' leadership in the family and structure role-play situations to motivate, elicit, and support parent competence.

> **W** = Watch the child and the parent carefully and redirect the role-play if needed.

> **E** = Empathize with all family members included in the role-play session to ensure mutual understanding, kindness, and respect.

> **R** = Review successes of role-plays and clarify how to apply targeted skills and corrective feedback to similar situations in the future.

When role-play is successful, change in the family is punctuated in that parent, and child behavior becomes more constructive in problem situations. The parent can also learn more about the child's perspective, appreciate the child's potential for learning new skills, and feel hope and motivation for a more positive family environment.

THEORY OF BEHAVIOR CHANGE

A key feature of the intervention approach for the Everyday Parenting curriculum is that it is model driven rather than a "school of therapy." Model-driven therapy is unique in that the target of change is defined by longitudinal data on the development of psychopathology (Dishion & Patterson, 1999). Thus it focuses on positive behavior support, healthy limits, and relationship building. In this approach, we integrate techniques of empirically supported interventions, such as acceptance and commitment therapy (Hayes, Strosahl, & Wilson, 1999), dialectical behavior therapy (Linehan, 2000), motivational interviewing (Miller & Rollnick, 2002), behavior analysis (Bijou, 1993), and cognitive-behavioral therapy (Kazdin, 1995). The science of clinical change, as of this writing, is underdeveloped, and it would be shortsighted to ignore the richness of intervention strategies found effective for addressing both adult and child behavior. Undoubtedly there is high potential for integrating and synthesizing interventions that are effective across a variety of client populations and, moreover, across psychopathologies and emotional disorders (Barlow, 2004).

We have devised empirically based hypotheses about interacting with clients and expected change. Much of this work is based on research about client resistance in behavioral approaches to supportive family change. Work by Patterson and Forgatch (1985) reveals a functional relationship between therapist behavior and client outcomes. More recently, Forgatch, Patterson, and DeGarmo (2005) documented an empirical relationship among therapists' display of knowledge of family management skills, skills in structuring sessions and meetings with caregivers to promote motivation and engagement, teaching and feedback skills, and motivation process skills. The general principle underlying the Everyday Parenting intervention model is to prioritize intervention services to address family management practices and to secondarily address other disruptive factors relevant to family management. As parenting skill is influenced by other factors, so, too, does parenting influence those factors. A focus on parenting is central to this model of intervention post-feedback. Family management is clearly the most beneficial factor in the reduction of mental health and behavioral health problems among all family members. This perspective is summarized in Figure 5.

From the work of Forgatch and colleagues, we know that children and families benefit from careful adherence to intervention dynamics that promote change in family management. There are four domains of therapist–client interaction that we particularly attend to in our work with families. The first (C) is **conceptual adherence** to the intervention model, which focuses on promoting behavioral health in families by targeting family management. Interventions that promote family management are prioritized over those that address mental health or disrupt contextual factors. The second factor (O) is to be **observant** and sensitive to client concerns and (A) **actively structure** sessions to promote optimal behavior change for the family. This involves prioritizing client–therapist discussions to avoid sidetracking and to focus on family management. The third factor (C) is to **carefully give feedback** and teach new skills. We know from therapist–client process research that indiscriminate teaching actually decreases clients' motivation to change. Teaching

FIGURE 5   **Family management in relation to other relevant factors.**

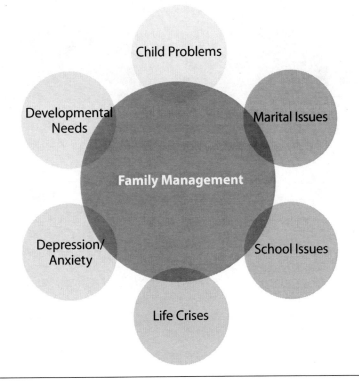

or providing feedback in a sensitive way involves validation and support, but it is also tailored according to a good interpersonal understanding of the needs and styles of each client. The fourth factor (H) is to provide **hope and motivation** in the service of promoting parenting change. The four domains comprise the COACH measure, which we developed (Dishion et al., 2010) to measure and support intervention fidelity while using the FCU and while implementing the Everyday Parenting intervention. Feedback about fidelity is used to increase the effectiveness of the intervention and to improve outcomes for families—a double reward for those engaged in the sometimes arduous role of family therapist. The hypothesized link between therapist performance and client change is shown in Figure 6.

As previously discussed, in this model the intervention needs of families are addressed across the continuum of adjustment. For example, some families may require less-intensive interventions given their many parenting strengths and may perhaps benefit from only brief, supportive interventions. Others may clearly require more intensive support as they change their parenting practices, perhaps multiple meetings per week, as is the approach of multisystemic family therapy (Henggeler & Lee, 2003; Henggeler, Schoenwald, Borduin, Rowland, & Cunningham, 1998). The Everyday Parenting curriculum, then, is appropriate for services ranging from prevention to treatment of serious mental health problems in children and adolescents, including those in residential or foster care settings in which it is critical to provide support

FIGURE 6   Parenting change process: The COACH model.

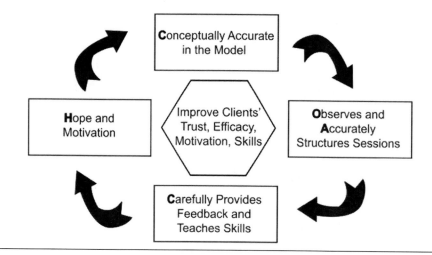

to caregivers during and following treatment. The Everyday Parenting curriculum is compatible with the PMTO and the Multidimensional Treatment Foster Care model, both of which emerged from the pioneering work at OSLC (Chamberlain & Moore, 1998; Forgatch, Patterson, & DeGarmo, 2005; Patterson, 1974).

SUMMARY

This curriculum provides a step-by-step guide to support caregivers while they are improving their everyday parenting practices. The overall approach is unique with respect to being assessment driven, motivational, developmentally flexible, tailored, and adaptive. It is also unique in that it addresses the needs of families across the range of service needs, from prevention to treatment of disrupted family systems and treatment of child or adolescent psychopathology and problem behavior.

Positive Behavior Support

Parent Requests and Child Cooperation

OVERVIEW AND RATIONALE

This session builds the foundation for enhancing parents' use of positive behavior support with their children or adolescents. The term *positive behavior support* comes from research on effective teaching and parenting. It is the practice of prompting and reinforcing positive youth behavior in an effort to decrease behavior problems, support children's skill development, and promote confidence and well-being. The first step in building positive behavior support is to change how parents think about children's problem behavior. By turning a negative label for a behavior into a specific positive goal, parents can teach, prompt, and offer positive behavior support through reinforcement. For example, instead of describing a child as "lazy," parents can offer a positive goal: the child cooperates with requests to help around the house. When families are in distress, however, it may be challenging for them to let go of global negative labels and to engage in the hopeful process of making positive behavior changes daily.

Coercion is a common experience in distressed families. When it gets out of hand, coercion can cause parents' and children's interactions to escalate into conflict or, worse, cause parents to avoid dealing with their child or adolescent. Some issues can develop into more-serious mental health problems. Many parents feel like giving up on trying to make a difference in their child's or adolescent's life. This response is usually a sign that coercion has taken its toll on parent motivation.

The first step a parent takes in the coercion cycle is to react emotionally to the child's problem behavior. When a behavior upsets parents, they may do one of several things: completely avoid discussing the situation and be angry, do something to hurt the youth (yelling, hitting, name calling), or make requests or demands that are unclear, blaming, or unrealistic and that lead to more conflict. Figure 7 offers a model of our work with parents to support

FIGURE 7   *Top:* **How coercion works to disrupt family interactions.** *Bottom:* **How a successful intervention can support family management.**

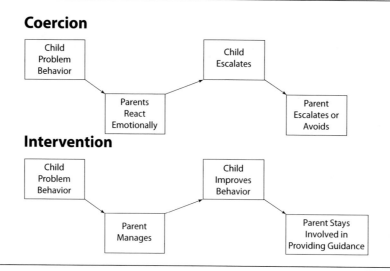

their management of the situation, which often means being aware of their own emotional reactions and regulating these emotions to guide the child to improved behavior through effective requests. This response requires mindfulness, some level of planning, and being realistic about the situation and the youth's abilities.

There are several possible benefits to parents and youths of practicing positive behavior support on a daily basis: (1) family relationships improve and conflict decreases; (2) youths develop competence in cooperation, self-regulation, and other prosocial skills; (3) parents gain a sense of self-efficacy in parenting; and (4) parents and the youth both gain an improved sense of well-being. Because opportunities for parents to make requests and for youths to respond to requests occur daily, a change from either an avoidant or a coercive approach to a healthy, positive approach can have very significant effects on the life of the family.

SUGGESTED TOOLS

➤ Videotaped examples of skillful, positive requests that are developmentally appropriate

➤ Tracking form for parent requests and youth cooperation

➤ Family observation video from the Family Check-Up assessment

➤ Whiteboard, chalkboard, or large sheets of paper

SESSION OBJECTIVES

➤ Parents should understand the principle underlying the importance of making requests or directives that are clear, specific, realistic, respectful, and noncoercive.

➤ Parents are able to discriminate between an effective request and an ineffective request (one that is unlikely to lead to child cooperation or that will escalate conflict).

➤ Parents practice making positive requests in a role-play and with their child at home.

➤ Parents clearly define what constitutes the child's cooperation with parent requests.

➤ Parents are shown how to track requests and cooperation between sessions.

COMMON PITFALLS AND SOLUTIONS

Motivation

When children do not cooperate with parents' requests, the parents tend to see the behavior as the child's problem rather than examine their own ways of making the requests. Furthermore, the parent may be afraid to make a direct request of a child because of the reaction of the child or of another family member, as can happen when parenting roles are conflicted or unclear. While motivating parents to change how they perceive and respond to problem behavior, it is important that the therapist help the parent anticipate the potential motivational barriers, offer support, and discuss and role-play solutions that tailor the intervention realistically to the family.

Tailoring

The key issue in tailoring this skill is using examples that are relevant to the parents' specific concerns and linking them to the youth's cooperation. The coercion diagram shown in Figure 7 can be used as a framework for relating specific examples of the parents' interactions with their child. While teaching skills, it is also helpful to use language that fits the family's cultural orientation and educational level. For example, using the terms *directives* or *commands* with parents who are uncomfortable with the term *requests* will help them better learn and incorporate the skill into their parenting. There are some major differences in how the coercion cycle plays out with children and with adolescents, so the examples should be adapted to the developmental level of the child. When parents are unaware that they are avoiding making requests because of past conflict, role-playing will be a helpful strategy to support their self-efficacy in the future when they make requests, manage conflict, and elicit child cooperation.

Structuring Sessions to Reduce Barriers

Based on results from the Family Check-Up, the therapist often has a sense of the barriers that parents may experience when it comes to making direct, clear, and effective requests of their child. Common barriers to making effective requests are linked to motivational problems as described earlier, to family situations with unclear roles, to parent depression or avoidance, and other situations. The therapist can support parents by anticipating these barriers and tailoring content and especially role-play to address or avoid barriers. For example, with a recently blended family, the therapist may want to structure role-plays so that the biological parent rather than the new stepparent is the one to initially make requests for behavior change. The stepparent can be assigned a more supportive role, for example. In this way, the therapist structures the session toward a family interaction pattern that will avoid potential conflict and motivational barriers.

> ### Note
> Blocks of italicized text are used to distinguish therapist statements from instructions and other text. The therapist statements used throughout this book are provided as examples and guidelines for use in counseling sessions.

SETTING THE AGENDA

Good to see you again. Have there been any issues or events since the time we did the feedback session?

Listen, support, and link to the agenda today, but avoid questions that open up topics that are not relevant to where you want to go with this family (e.g., "How's the job going?" "How is your depression?" "Have you been taking care of yourself?").

It sounds like a lot has happened since we last talked. Let's talk more about those things at the end of our meeting today. I had planned to get started on our work together to [get Chris to be cooperative]. Does that still sound like a good plan for you?

In your feedback meeting, we decided that you would like to work on improving [Chris's] behavior and on your abilities to provide positive support.

If you don't mind, to make sure that I'm helpful in moving us forward, I made a plan for our meeting today to help us stay on track. I planned that we would cover the following today (write on a piece of paper, white-board, etc., so the parent can see the list):

• What positive behavior support is

• Turning a negative into a positive behavior

• Making clear and effective requests

• Identifying and planning around barriers

• Home practice experiments

Does this seem doable? You can see that we have a fair amount to do today to get you started. I would like to comment that this is how I will usually work with you, in that you and I will set the agenda before each session so you will have input into what we talk about. Our focus will be on getting through the family management tools that you identified in the Family Check-Up. Each of our meetings will include a family management skill and a communication skill. I will also suggest a home practice exercise to give you a chance to see how these things work at home with your family.

WHAT IS POSITIVE BEHAVIOR SUPPORT?

All children can present challenges to adults from time to time. Young children challenge parents with behaviors such as tantrums, fighting, and whining. Teenagers challenge parents by being defiant and by engaging in problem behavior, such as lying. Teen behavior can be challenging because it often occurs outside the home and is difficult for parents to observe or even know about.

Regardless of the situation, how you react to problem behavior can make things worse or better. Research has shown that it's the daily patterns that can get parents into trouble. Our focus on family management and communication is an effort to improve how you handle the day-to-day behaviors of your child.

To start the process, a tool that most parents find helpful is turning a negative behavior into a positive one. I'd like you to, first, take a step back and think about what you would like to see **more of** *rather than what you want to see* **less of**. *This will give you a positive base to work from.*

FAMILY MANAGEMENT SKILL: PINPOINTING POSITIVE BEHAVIORS

To be successful, start small. To help a child learn a positive behavior, it's important to break it down into the small steps of the positive behavior. Small behaviors can be more easily observed and rewarded. For example, if you want to change your child's neatness level, one small step to start with is "pick things up off the floor." That's an easy step to see and to encourage.

Pinpointing is a way to identify positive behaviors. Increasing positive behavior naturally decreases negative behavior. As a result, increasing positive behavior is the easiest way to begin.

Let's look at an example from Handout 1A. This is about having problems getting up and getting ready for school in the morning.

Pinpointing a behavior gives you a good idea about the steps involved in making a positive behavior change. You can get information about how well your child is doing with each of the steps by tracking them on a daily basis.

FAMILY COMMUNICATION SKILL: MAKING EFFECTIVE AND CLEAR REQUESTS

The second tool is giving directions to your child in a way that ensures [she] is as clear as you are about what is expected of [her]. Sound simple? Well, it isn't that simple and usually requires practice. This is the first step of positive behavior support for your child.

As you probably know, a lot can go wrong when you give a direction. For instance, requests that are too complicated or that show disapproval, criticize, or blame are unlikely to lead to cooperation and generally fall in the category of making things worse.

Let's take a look at Handout 1B, which describes behaviors to avoid and skills that can help you make requests that your [child or teen] will follow.

Remaining neutral doesn't always come naturally when talking with children, but it's really important if you want your child to cooperate. Let's practice staying neutral while making effective requests.

Wrong Way/Right Way for Requests

Wrong way: "Why don't you ever help in the kitchen?"

Right way: _____

Wrong way: "Don't throw your books on the floor."

Right way: _____

Wrong way: "You're such a slob in the bathroom."

Right way: _____

Wrong way: "Things never change. You never take out the trash."

Right way: _____

ROLE-PLAY MAKING CLEAR AND EFFECTIVE REQUESTS

Provide parents with a lot of practice giving requests the right way. Practice sets them up for success in doing the home practice assignment—giving effective requests, tracking the way they give requests, and tracking their child's cooperation. Giving an effective request has three parts for the parent to practice:

1. Giving the request: "Put your backpack in the closet now, please."

2. Staying involved: Monitor to see that the child cooperates.

3. Noticing and praising cooperation: "Thank you for putting your backpack in the closet."

Today we'll focus just on making a request and also set you up to observe how much [Chris] cooperates when asked to do something.

To make sure you are successful when you practice at home, let's practice here in the session first. Let's start with the example of [you asking Chris to help more in the kitchen]. First, I'd like to be [Chris], and you use one of the wrong ways to make a request shown on Handout 1B.

Great! Now let's try the right way.

Role-play making requests, taking turns using the wrong way and the right way. Role-play actively engages parents in the learning process and highlights the key behaviors to use and to avoid when making requests.

FAMILY MANAGEMENT SKILL: TRACKING DAILY BEHAVIOR

It is hard to know how best to change family management without observing a problem behavior carefully. Tracking means keeping a record of what you'd like to change. Tracking is important because it helps you notice changes in your own behavior and your child's behavior. The information you gather helps you see if things are improving, staying the same, or getting worse. Parents are often surprised what they find out by tracking.

Let's look at an example on the Session 1 Tracking Form on Handout 1C. This time, tracking will focus on two things: (1) effective requests you make and (2) whether or not your child cooperates with those requests.

The form is designed to keep track of the primary behavior you want to change, which is noncooperation with your requests. The form will also enable you to keep track of how you gave your request in the first place. Was your tone neutral, or was it not neutral?

Noncooperation with adults is at the core of most problem behavior in children at home and at school. The goal of a request is to encourage cooperation. We often don't know how frequently our children cooperate with requests. The first step in behavior change is to assess how things are working in your family. That means that this week you will track both the kinds of requests you make and your child's cooperation.

Tip

Take parents through the blank form, explaining the definition of *co-operation*—starting to do what parents ask within 15 seconds—and how to mark cooperation or noncooperation. Give parents plenty of time to ask questions. Some parents may disagree with the need for the child to cooperate the first time the request is made. Explain that to avoid arguments and repeat requests, prompt cooperation works best. Another point of discussion could be that 15 seconds is not long enough. Typically, if you ask a parent to make a request, then time 15 seconds, parents will see that this is more than enough time for children to comply.

Since you're practicing requests, this will be a good opportunity to observe the number of times your child is cooperating with your wishes.

To make tracking your child's behavior a little easier, decide on the time of day that you can pay attention and are able to observe. Good times to track are transition times or times that you would typically make requests, such as morning routines, after school, after dinner, or just before bed. Decide on a place to keep the form so you know where it is. Tracking your child's behavior as many days as possible during the week will help give you a good picture of your child's cooperation.

It's also important to explain to your child that you're doing a tracking exercise before you begin. Let [her] know that you will fill out this form during the week as part of your practice. The goal of the activity is to gather information, so don't expect that you'll see many changes this next week. You'll learn a lot simply by recording what usually happens.

HOME PRACTICE

This week, I encourage you to track how your child cooperates with your requests. I'd like you to keep track of the requests you make of your child. Were the requests effective or not effective? How did your child respond to your requests? Complete the Session 1 Tracking Form on Handout 1D.

HOME PRACTICE OUTLINE

1. Track how your child complies with your requests.

2. On the tracking form, record how you handled making the request.

Example

Problem behavior: Late for school, irresponsible

Positive: Get ready for school in the morning means:

1. Getting up when the alarm rings.

2. Being dressed by a certain time.

3. Eating breakfast.

4. Organizing school materials.

Now let's use that example to complete the following activity. In each case, we turn a problem into a teaching opportunity for children and adolescents. Below are some common problems. Pinpoint some positive behaviors that would help change the problem.

Problem behavior: Lawanda never cleans her room.

Positive: Cleaning her room means:

1. Making her bed.

2. _____

3. _____

Problem behavior: Amy grabs toys from her older brother.

Positive: Playing nicely includes:

1. Asking nicely for a toy.

2. Waiting until it's her turn to play.

3. _____

Problem behavior: Jerome has problems with schoolwork.

Positive: Schoolwork includes:

1. Bringing homework home.

2. _____

3. _____

Problem: Devon is always yelling at or fighting with his older sister.

Positive: Getting along with his sister includes:

1. Talking in a normal tone of voice.

2. _____

3. _____

Behaviors to Avoid When Making Positive Requests

Blaming, criticizing, or showing disapproval: "It's your fault this house is a mess."

Asking a question: "Do you want to clean your room?"

Making too many requests at once: "Clean your room, wash the dishes, and do your homework."

Bringing up side issues: "Your grades stink. Now clean your room."

Bringing up ancient history: "You've always been sloppy. Remember the time …?"

Yelling from a distance: "Get over here right now and get your shoes on!"

Making Requests That Work

What to Do

Be specific.

Make only one request at a time.

Focus on what you want, not what you don't want: "Please put the dishes away now."

How to Do It

Use a pleasant but firm tone.

Keep your facial expression neutral.

Make eye contact.

Be polite and respectful.

Follow through—see that the child does what is asked.

Notice when child cooperates: "Thank you for putting your dishes away."

From *Everyday Parenting: A Professional's Guide to Building Family Management Skills,* © 2012 by T. J. Dishion, E. A. Stormshak, and K. A. Kavanagh, Champaign, IL: Research Press (www.researchpress.com, 800-519-2707).

HANDOUT 1C

Session 1 Tracking Form (Completed Example)

Give three examples of a request you made (effective or not effective) and what your child did (i.e., cooperated or did not cooperate).

Behavior change area (specify behavior and date to be completed): _____ cooperation; by June 9_____

	Sun. + Effective – Not effective	Mon. + Effective – Not effective	Tues. + Effective – Not effective	Wed. + Effective – Not effective	Thurs. + Effective – Not effective	Fri. + Effective – Not effective	Sat. + Effective – Not effective
Parent made request (+ or –)	+ – +	+ + +	+ +	– + +	– – –	+ +	+ + + +
Child cooperated (+ or –)	+ + –	– – –	+ +	– + +	+ – –	+ +	+ – – +

Time of tracking: _____6:00_____ A.M. (P.M) to _____9:00_____ A.M (P.M)

From *Everyday Parenting: A Professional's Guide to Building Family Management Skills*, © 2012 by T.J. Dishion, E.A. Stormshak, and K.A. Kavanagh, Champaign, IL: Research Press (www.researchpress.com, 800-519-2707).

HANDOUT 1D

Give three examples of a request you made (effective or not effective) and what your child did (i.e., cooperated or did not cooperate).

Behavior change area (specify behavior and date to be completed): _____

	Sun.		Mon.		Tues.		Wed.		Thurs.		Fri.		Sat.	
Request was	+ Effective	− Not effective	+ Effective	− Not effective	+ Effective	− Not effective	+ Effective	− Not effective	+ Effective	− Not effective	+ Effective	− Not effective	+ Effective	− Not effective
Parent made request (+ or −)														
Child cooperated (+ or −)														

Time of tracking: _____ A.M./P.M. to _____ A.M./P.M.

Positive Behavior Support

Parent Praise for Positive Behavior

OVERVIEW AND RATIONALE

This session focuses on motivating parents to increase the density of their skillful use of praise for positive child behavior by labeling ("I see you put the trash out when I asked!") and by using praise to show appreciation and to reinforce positive behavior ("Great job!" or "That helps!").

The rationale for focusing on this family management practice is that increasing parents' verbal support for children's positive behavior has two outcomes. First, it strengthens the youth's positive behavior through reinforcement. Second, and equally important, verbal praise and incentives for positive behavior reduce the likelihood of coercive interaction patterns. When the level of reinforcement increases in a family, the incentive for negative child behavior decreases.

This simple yet fundamental change in family interaction is captured in the functional assessment of child behavior, or the ABCs of behavior. All family interactions have an antecedent (A), a behavior (B), and a consequence (C). When all three steps are positive, it creates the ABCs of the positive family change cycle (see Figure 8). Antecedents occur before a behavior and set the stage for success or failure. An effective request (A), for example, sets the stage for youth cooperation (B), which leads to a reward, such as praise (C). Examples of antecedents that are unlikely to be successful include parents yelling unspecific and critical demands ("I told you to help around here!"). Effective requests, on the other hand, are more likely to lead to success ("Please take out the trash now"). The behavior that follows is either cooperative (positive) or argumentative ("I did it yesterday!"). The focus of this session is on how the parents react to cooperation to build a positive change cycle in the family. Simply saying "great job" can increase the chances of child cooperation in the future and can give the parents confidence about their own family leadership.

FIGURE 8   The ABCs of positive family change.

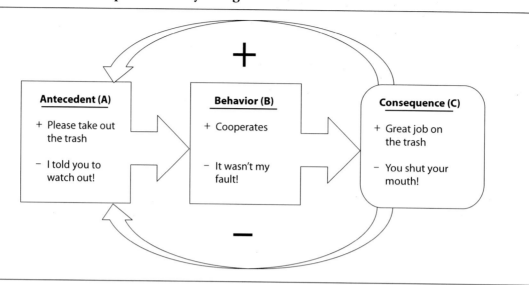

The goal of this session is to increase the parents' use of personal and verbal reinforcement. Given that all children and adults benefit from reinforcement to maintain positive behaviors and, more important, to learn new behaviors, praise and positive reinforcement is a vital skill for parents to learn. A general principle to follow is a minimum reinforcement-to-correction ratio of 4:1; that is, four praises to one correction. Thus the goal of this session is to increase the density of *contingent* positive reinforcement and praise from the parent. Although unconditional love and positive regard are the foundation of all healthy relationships, to help parents increase their leadership role in teaching new behaviors, it is essential that they learn to use praise as a consequence for positive and skillful child behavior.

The ABCs of family interaction occur daily in all families, and the vast majority are unintended side effects of family living. It is a fact of daily family life that much of what we say and do is unconscious and automatic. It is typical to notice the negative and expect the positive. So parents and caregivers may not be aware that they rarely praise or notice their child's positive behavior. Another common problem occurs when the form of praise parents use is actually experienced by the adolescent as negative because it is accompanied by blame or criticism. The first step in raising awareness of this pattern can occur during feedback as part of the Family Check-Up. The second step in building and motivating change involves using role-play and watching videos on effective requests and verbal support.

It is also quite common that parents' preoccupation and ignoring is an antecedent to a problem behavior. When parents refocus their attention on the child's activities, they may realize that he or she is not behaving as expected. An emotional response to the situation is likely to make things worse. What is needed to correct the situation is to provide an effective request that is realistic for the child; for example, "Oops, we didn't put paper down before you started to paint. Please stop right now and go wipe your hands off." When the child returns with clean hands the parent says, "Ah, yes, thank you for washing your hands. Now let's put paper underneath so you can paint some more." When parents realize their own lack of attentiveness is truly the antecedent to a problem behavior, they can correct the course and keep moving forward in a positive change cycle.

The family assessment identifies the major patterns of parents' responses to positive and negative child behaviors. If you are offering sessions on positive behavior support, you have already had a discussion with the parents about the need to further develop and practice reinforcement for positive behavior. Note that many parents have this skill in their repertoire but fail to use it in their parenting or close family relationships. This is a point of discussion and can be related to how an adult was raised, to a history of conflict in the family, and/or to a parent's comfort level with being supportive rather than correcting and setting limits. Parental stress and depression are other contextual issues that can make praising difficult. If discussion during the Family Check-Up has revealed that a family is dealing with these challenges, they should be discussed and anticipated in role-plays.

SUGGESTED TOOLS

➤ Videotaped examples of skillful verbal support that are developmentally appropriate for the targeted child

➤ Tracking form with parent requests, youth cooperation, and praise

➤ Family observation video from the Family Check-Up assessment

➤ Whiteboard, chalkboard, or large sheets of paper

SESSION OBJECTIVES

➤ Parents will understand and appreciate the importance of praise and verbal support in their own families.

➤ Parents are able to give skillful verbal support that is developmentally appropriate for their child.

➤ Parents are able to identify their own barriers to praise and verbal support.

➤ Parents are shown how to track requests and cooperation and to practice giving praise.

➤ Parents are shown how to track pinpointed goal behavior.

COMMON PITFALLS AND SOLUTIONS

Motivation

Most parents agree that it is important to praise their child, but they may differ about when and for what behaviors. ("Why should I praise her for doing what is expected?" or "I was never praised for helping around the house, I just did it.") A related issue is a long-standing conflict or a negative history between a parent and child. Parents who are holding a grudge or are feeling defeated may find it difficult to praise a child. A third issue is that parents slip subtle or not-so-subtle criticism into praise. We call them *zaps*, which dilute the power of the parents' praise ("At least you are showing up for school. That's a change!").

Tailoring

The therapist needs to understand the dynamics of the parent and child relationship and to gather information on the history of praise and levels of existing conflicts. In addition, the therapist should ask about the ease and difficulty of parents giving praise and about the child's responses to praise. On occasion, parents may be encouraged to act as if there is no history of negative interaction for a week to see how things change if they praise, even though it may not come from deep inside.

Structuring Sessions to Reduce Barriers

It is suggested that barriers to contingent praise be discussed up front in this session. One self-assessment exercise that often helps motivate parents to praise is the exercise called "Messages from the Past and for the Future." If the proper time is taken, this exercise can be a powerful motivational tool. A more intensive structuring strategy has been in vivo visualization, during which parents lie down and the therapist takes the parents through a series of visualizations of themselves and their child in a setting, such as walking down the beach in the present, a year from now, 5 years from now, and 10 years in the future. How can parents help their child realize his or her potential? What aspect of their son or daughter would they like to bring to the forefront to help him or her be successful and happy?

SETTING THE AGENDA

Good to see you again. Let's see, last week we worked on making effective requests and just observing [Chris's] tendency to cooperate with the requests you made. Before we begin, has anything happened since the last time we met that I should know about before we move forward?

If anything has happened that would affect the parents' skill development during the session, it should be briefly addressed, and they should be asked if they are ready to continue the work started in the previous session.

I have planned that we would cover the following activities today (write on a piece of paper, whiteboard, etc., so the parents can see the list):

• Review home practice, troubleshooting.

• Do a brief exercise on family messages.

- Discuss giving [Chris] praise or support for cooperation with requests.

- Discuss the home practice experiments.

Does this seem doable for today? Is there anything else you would like to address?

Be responsive to the parents' concerns. Or tailor the list by adding items such as *two parents using praise* if you want to deal with a family dynamic in which only one parent acknowledges a child's behavior and you feel this could change.

Last session, we practiced making effective requests and tracking child co-operation. These skills set the foundation for positive family change. We'll review each of them before moving on to this session's skills. Positive verbal support is our family communication skill this session. Then we'll begin to figure out the positive behaviors you'd like your child to develop to replace the behaviors you see as problems.

REVIEW OF SESSION 1

Your home practice last week was to track your child's behavior and the requests you made to your child (effective or not effective) and whether your child complied or did not comply. Let's talk about what you learned from tracking these behaviors.

It's important to look at the parents' tracking sheet, if they have brought it, and to discuss the information on the sheet. This shows interest and builds collaboration in terms of the work parents are doing at home. If the parents haven't brought their tracking sheet, then asking the following questions is helpful.

QUESTIONS TO ASK PARENTS

➤ How many days did you track?

➤ What did you find out about your child's behavior?

➤ Did you see a relationship between how you made a request and your child's cooperation?

➤ Was there anything that made tracking hard for your family?

➤ What did you learn about yourself or your child from this week's tracking?

➤ Were there any antecedents, or things happening before, for you or your child that you observed that were particularly interesting?

PARENT SELF-ASSESSMENT: MESSAGES FROM THE PAST AND FOR THE FUTURE

Growing up, we're given a lot of messages about who we are and what we can do from adults who play a significant role in our lives (such as parents, caregivers, teachers, and coaches). While the exact words and situations might escape you, you probably retained the message behind the words. During the next week, take a few minutes to complete this activity. Think back about the messages you remember from your parents or caregivers that most influenced how you think about yourself and your capabilities today. Write those down.

Now think about what kinds of messages you are giving [Chris] about who [she] is and what you see in [her] future. Write down those messages and we'll discuss them in our review next session.

Messages from the past: *What messages were you given as a child about who you were and what you were capable of that, through either acceptance or resistance, have guided your self-image?*

Messages for the future: *What messages are you presently giving [Chris] about who [she] is and what you see in [her] future?*

FAMILY COMMUNICATION SKILL: PRAISE

Now we're going to talk about positive statements we can make to our children. Positive verbal support or praise is a way to let children know when we like what they're doing. If you kept track for 24 hours straight, you might be surprised at all the good things [Chris] does in a day. Of course, this isn't possible, but it is possible to catch [her] doing the right thing many times during a day. These moments are opportunities to give your child praise and increase the chances of [her] repeating the positive behavior.

Unfortunately, sometimes we're so busy, stressed, frustrated, or tired that we miss these opportunities. Often, we're so on the alert for problem behaviors that we overlook the good behavior. Even watching a TV show quietly for an hour may be a positive child behavior when you're tired. Letting your child know that the quiet hour was appreciated will make [her] feel good.

Giving praise can be as easy as saying thank you for something you appreciate. Focus on giving praise and not on your child's reaction to the praise. Whether they show it or not, most children like to be praised. Being specific helps your child know exactly what you like about [her] behavior. For example, "I really like it when you play so nicely with your little sister and share your things." Being specific helps children know the behaviors you want to see. If your praise is accompanied by a hug, a pat on the back, or a smile, it's more likely you will see these behaviors again.

Another effective way of giving praise is to tell someone important to your child, [her] grandmother or grandfather, for example, about [her] positive behavior. In some communities, it is very common to praise a child by telling a story to others about [his or her] positive behavior.

Let's review a list of some things we can say to let our kids know we like what they're doing. You'll probably think of things that aren't on the list, and we can add them to our handout as we go along.

Handout 2A lists examples of giving your child encouragement and increasing the likelihood that [she'll] repeat positive behavior. You can write down your own example from interactions with your child this week.

PRAISE AND ACKNOWLEDGMENT

➤ Make it simple: "Thank you."

➤ Do it right away.

➤ Be specific: "Very neat work on your report."

Encourage behavior or acts you would like to see repeated.

To give you a little practice, let's look at other parents' attempts at praise and do them the right way.

Wrong Way/Right Way for Praise

Wrong way: "Looks like you tried to help in the kitchen!"

Right way: _____

Wrong way: "The books made it halfway to your room!"

Right way: _____

Wrong way: "For once you picked up a towel."

Right way: _____

Wrong way: "Hey, it's a miracle—he said please!"

Right way: _____

ROLE-PLAY GIVING PRAISE AND VERBAL SUPPORT

Provide parents with a lot of practice giving appropriate, contingent praise tailored to the developmental level of the child. This helps them practice the ABCs of developing the positive behaviors you discussed in your last session. Practice sets them up for success in doing the home practice assignment— giving effective requests (antecedent), tracking the way they give the requests and their child's cooperation (behavior), and then acknowledging cooperation through praise (consequence).

TRACKING AND PRAISING PINPOINTED BEHAVIORS

This week you'll continue tracking your requests and your child's cooperation. Remember the skills we practiced last week for making effective requests? They're on Handout 1B and include being specific, making one request at a time, and focusing on what you want, not what you don't want. Also remember that it's important to use a pleasant but firm tone of voice, to keep your facial expression neutral, to make eye contact, and to be polite. Just like last time, to make tracking a little easier, decide on a time of day that you'll track (morning, after school, after dinner, before bed), and decide on a place to keep the tracking form so you know where it is. In addition to tracking cooperation, we are going to start working on realizing the goal that you set in the first session when we turned your concern for [Chris] into a positive goal.

This week you'll fill out the blank tracking form (Handout 2C) with the pinpointed behaviors that make up your positive goal, and you can use the examples that we went over last time as a guide. You will use your skills in making effective requests for each of the pinpointed behaviors you identify and practice offering praise when each step is done.

There are two possible outcomes of your work these first 2 weeks. You may find that your child is more cooperative than usual or that you never realized how uncooperative your child really is. If the latter is the case, don't be discouraged. Your goal is to step back and gather information. On the other hand, if your child is more cooperative than usual, enjoy it. Sometimes there is a monitoring effect when you start tracking a child's behavior. These effects are often short lived. Next session, we'll focus on incentives that help maintain these positive behaviors we are working on.

Tip

Emphasize that this week is different from Session 1. Last session, parents were tracking requests and child cooperation. This time they also are tracking the positive behavior they wish to teach. Read through and explain the example in Handout 2B. In addition to tracking requests and child cooperation, positive behavior is defined, the time of tracking is identified, and the behavior is pinpointed—that is, broken down into clear, measurable steps. For skilled parents, have them complete the form at home. For families who need more help, complete the form together during the session. Also take parents through a role-play of requesting and praising one of the behaviors.

HOME PRACTICE OUTLINE

1. Continue tracking your requests and your child's cooperation for some period of time each day (15 minutes to an hour).

2. Track your child's completion of the pinpointed steps you've identified as those that will make a positive change in his or her behavior.

Examples of Praise and Encouragement

"You have improved in …"

"I like it when you …"

"Great job checking in after school."

"You've done a wonderful job of …"

"What a terrific idea …"

"Good for you for …"

"You are doing so well."

"That was a good decision."

"You showed a lot of maturity when you …"

"Look how well you did …"

"What a wonderful job you've done with …"

"That's a really interesting way to …"

"It pleases me when you …"

"That's a perfect way to …"

"I'm so happy you …"

"Thank you for …"

"That's terrific—you got all your homework done."

"Thanks for being so responsible and getting home on time."

"What a nice job of …"

"Hey, you are really sharp! You …"

"I really appreciate you doing your chores without a reminder."

"That _____ was so nice."

"That's great! It looks beautiful."

"I'm very proud of you for …"

"How thoughtful of you to …"

"Beautiful!"

"Fine!"

"Great!"

"Fantastic!"

"Tremendous!"

"You should have seen [Chris] play today."

Examples of Physical Praise

A pat on the arm or shoulder

A hug

Gentle hair ruffle

Affectionate arm squeeze

A kiss

High-five

Thumbs-up

From *Everyday Parenting: A Professional's Guide to Building Family Management Skills,* © 2012 by T. J. Dishion, E. A. Stormshak, and K. A. Kavanagh, Champaign, IL: Research Press (www.researchpress.com, 800-519-2707).

HANDOUT 2B

Session 2 Tracking Form (Completed Example)

Give three examples of a request you made (effective or not effective) and what your child did (i.e., complied or did not comply).

Behavior Change Area: ___clean kitchen by 7:00 p.m.___

(Specify behavior and time to be completed.)

Pinpointed Behaviors	Sun. + Effective – Not effective	Mon. + Effective – Not effective	Tue. + Effective – Not effective	Wed. + Effective – Not effective	Thurs. + Effective – Not effective	Fri. + Effective – Not effective	Sat. + Effective – Not effective
Request was							
Put dishes in dishwasher	+	+	+	+	+	+	
Wash pans	+	+	+		+	–	
Wipe off counters	+	+	+	–	+		
Sweep floor	–		+		+	+	

Effective Request/Cooperation	Sun.	Mon.	Tue.	Wed.	Thurs.	Fri.	Sat.
Parent made request	+ + +	+	+ +	+ + +		+ + + +	+ +
Child cooperated	+ + +	O	+ +	+ +		+ + +	

Time of tracking: __7:00__ A.M.(P.M) to __8:00__ A.M.(P.M)

From *Everyday Parenting: A Professional's Guide to Building Family Management Skills*, © 2012 by T. J. Dishion, E. A. Stormshak, and K. A. Kavanagh, Champaign, IL: Research Press (www.researchpress.com, 800-519-2707).

Give three examples of a request you made (effective or not effective) and what your child did (i.e., complied or did not comply).

Behavior Change Area: _____

(Specify behavior and time to be completed.)

Pinpointed Behaviors	Sun.	Mon.	Tue.	Wed.	Thurs.	Fri.	Sat.
Request was	+ Effective – Not effective	+ Effective – Not effective	+ Effective – Not effective	+ Effective – Not effective	+ Effective – Not effective	+ Effective – Not effective	+ Effective – Not effective
Put dishes in dishwasher							
Wash pans							
Wipe off counters							
Sweep floor							

Effective Request/Cooperation	Sun.	Mon.	Tue.	Wed.	Thurs.	Fri.	Sat.
Parent made request							
Child cooperated							

Time of tracking: _____ A.M./P.M. to _____ A.M./P.M.

From *Everyday Parenting: A Professional's Guide to Building Family Management Skills*, © 2012 by T. J. Dishion, E. A. Stormshak, and K. A. Kavanagh, Champaign, IL: Research Press (www.researchpress.com, 800-519-2707).

Behavior-Change Plans

Instruction and Incentives

OVERVIEW AND RATIONALE

A central theme in positive behavior support is to develop realistic behavior-change plans that include contingent incentives. Behavior-change plans use unwanted behavior as an opportunity to teach youths important new skills, such as doing daily chores and homework. Effective behavior-change plans require a proactive approach to prompt children's positive behavior and to mindfully react to children's successes from day to day. Parents' ability to monitor themselves and the reactions and behavior of their child is central to effective behavior-change plans. This session focuses on defining the features of successful incentives for children, creating a behavior-change plan that fits the family, and practicing presenting the behavior-change plan to children. Structured exercises for introducing the behavior-change plan to the child are provided.

The benefit to the child of a successful behavior-change plan is development of self-regulation, which is a strong resiliency factor in a variety of life circumstances. The value to the parent of a successful behavior-change plan is improved family atmosphere and increased parental self-efficacy.

The first step, as we discussed in the first session, is to restate the issue, changing it from a problem behavior into a teachable positive behavior. For example, name calling can be recast as *needing to be respectful*. If children are fighting with siblings, introducing a good-behavior game can provide incentives for 10 minutes of respectful behavior by the siblings, which essentially means 10 minutes of no name calling. If this intervention is successful, then the children will have learned to regulate their own emotional reactions that lead to fighting, and the parent will feel more confident that he or she can function as a leader in the family. Another example of using a behavior-change plan is to teach a child or adolescent a more complicated skill, such as doing a chore (cleaning up the kitchen daily). Although it is often assumed that teenagers know what we mean when we ask them to clean up the kitchen, they often do not. Cleaning up the kitchen involves a series of tasks, such as putting away the dishes, wiping down the counters, and cleaning up trash. Providing this level of detail to adolescents and using praise and incentives will help the child develop the skills to clean up the kitchen and will thus reduce conflict. Then, most important, chores are done daily with less prompting, cajoling, or criticism from the parent.

A third example of the use of a behavior-change plan involves promoting a homework routine, which could include making a place in the house that is quiet and free from distractions for doing homework, organizing and keeping track of homework, withholding rewarding activities until homework is completed, and the like. Homework is a complex skill that can be challenging for some parents who never cultivated this skill in themselves. Helping parents successfully develop homework routines has many benefits to the child. Children's ability to do homework regularly is highly predictive of academic success.

The central idea in successful behavior-change plans is shaping positive child behavior. This simply means that we start with the skill level of the child or adolescent and then in the following weeks shape the youth's development of positive behavior and skill. When thinking about the process of instruction, we accept that as students we begin with the basics, and when we become skilled at them, we develop more complex skills (e.g., music, dance, martial arts, academic subjects). The same idea can be applied to everyday family interaction and child behavior. It is important to teach the basic behavior, then move to more complex behaviors.

Behavior-change plans such as point charts and behavior-change contracts seem simple enough, but they are in fact quite complicated to implement in day-to-day family life. There are two major mistakes that adults can make while implementing a behavior-change plan. One is having unrealistic behavior-change goals that ask for changes in themselves and their children that are far beyond their current skill levels. For example, in a family that is chaotic and busy, setting up a family chore chart with children doing 2 hours of chores a day is likely to fail, regardless of the incentives. Such a plan is too much of a stretch for all those concerned.

A second area of difficulty in implementing a behavior-change plan involves parents' consistency in using it. If the behavior-change plan is not implemented consistently, it will not be successful. Parents' own problems, such as depression or stress, may undermine consistency and limit other interpersonal behaviors that are important for caregiving. For a depressed parent, starting small and building success will be more useful than being overly ambitious. Parental depression is assessed in the Family Check-Up and should be discussed as part of background considerations while setting behavior-change goals. Thus a behavior-change plan is unrealistic if it is beyond the emotional capability or skill level of the parent. If this is a concern, it is best to address it with honesty and compassion. The goal of such a discussion is for parents to become more aware of how their own emotions and adjustment affect their parenting; this awareness in turn facilitates their collaboration while tailoring family management interventions that optimize success.

During the Family Check-Up, it is difficult to evaluate the parents' skill in implementing behavior change, partly because it involves a behavior that takes place over several days. However, it is possible to evaluate how proactive the parents are and the extent to which they monitor and track their children's behavior on a daily basis. Contextual issues such as stress, mental health, substance use and abuse, and marital difficulties can be barriers to proactive parenting and monitoring in general and to successful behavior-change plans specifically.

SUGGESTED TOOLS

➤ Videotaped examples of parent reviewing a point chart or behavior-change plan that is developmentally appropriate for the targeted child

➤ For a youth for whom homework is a concern, a videotape about homework skills

➤ Handout about achievable goals

➤ Behavior-change plan form that is developmentally appropriate for the child or adolescent and tailored to the child and family

➤ Whiteboard, chalkboard, or large sheets of paper

SESSION OBJECTIVES

➤ Secure parents' willingness to adopt realistic behavior-change goals.

➤ Parents are able to clearly instruct the child on the behavior-change plan to optimize the child's understanding and engagement.

➤ Parents are able to identify their own barriers to implementing a behavior-change plan and to providing contingent incentives.

➤ Parents are prepared for a successful behavior-change plan experiment for the next week.

COMMON PITFALLS AND SOLUTIONS

Motivation

Many of the barriers to changing the way parents use praise also are barriers to behavior-change plans. The major issue is helping parents discriminate between incentives and bribes. We include a section about this issue and offer discussion responses that will motivate parents to have a proactive plan for using incentives to teach and promote positive behavior in their children. The bottom line is that incentives are used in every family and occur every day, and we are helping parents be more mindful of contingencies that promote positive behavior and a more pleasant family atmosphere.

Tailoring

The child's age and developmental level are critical to the tailoring process. Many families have children who range in age from early childhood through adolescence, so behavior-change plans may have to be adjusted to be developmentally appropriate for each child. An adolescent may be functioning more at the age 7 to 8 level, so the therapist would need to tailor the behavior-change plan accordingly. It is also advisable to tailor the plan to the interest of the child or adolescent. At times it makes sense to interview the youth about possible incentives and to get his or her input about the intervention. Creativity is encouraged. For example, one therapist placed the child's photograph on a dollar bill and created "Jacob bucks," which were then photocopied and given to the child for completing 80% of his chores that day. A certain number of bucks could be exchanged for a range of incentives. This was a highly effective and positive intervention for Jacob and his mom.

Structuring Sessions to Reduce Barriers

It is important to address barriers to implementing a behavior-change plan, such as parents' emotional well-being, work schedules, and stress levels. If parents have a minimal educational background, behavior-change plans should be developed that have a minimum number of steps, and clear examples of accomplishing these steps should be discussed and role-played in session. At least half of the session time should be devoted to discussing the supports for and barriers to carrying out a behavior-change plan within the family. This not only helps a family to successfully carry out the plan, but it also works toward the long-term goal of families incorporating this strategy into family practices when new problem behaviors emerge. With respect to incentives, an honest discussion of the parents' resources to provide incentives and of their importance as a tool to encourage child participation is a fundamental part of this session. For those families with limited resources, the importance of praise and encouragement should be emphasized.

SETTING THE AGENDA

Good to see you again. Let's see, last week we worked on making effective requests and observing [Chris's] tendency to cooperate with the requests you made. Before we begin, has anything happened since the last time we met that I should know about before we move forward?

If anything has happened that would affect parents' skill development during the session, it should be briefly addressed, and they should be asked if they are ready to continue the work started in the previous session.

I have planned that we would cover the following today (write on a piece of paper, whiteboard, etc., so the parents can see the list):

- Review home practice, troubleshooting.

- Discuss setting up a behavior-change plan that uses incentives.

- Do exercises on giving your child instructions about the behavior-change plan.

- Discuss the home practice experiments.

Does this seem doable for today? Is there anything else you would like to address?

Be responsive to the parents' concerns. Or tailor the list by adding items such as *two parents using praise* if you want to deal with a family dynamic in which only one parent acknowledges a child's behavior and you feel this could change.

In this meeting, we are going to work on putting in place a behavior-change plan for making progress on your goal to [get Chris to do her homework every day]. This is a plan you can follow day to day to prompt and to motivate positive behavior. The plan is really as much for yourself as it is for [Chris]. Many parents will wonder why they need to change how they do things when their child has the problem. The way I like to think about this is that parents are teachers, and problem behavior is an opportunity or sign that your child needs to learn a new behavior or skill. You are the ones to guide that change.

REVIEW OF SESSION 2

Last session, we talked about messages from the past and positive verbal support. You also tracked your behavior and your child's behavior during the week.

So far, you've been collecting information about your behavior and your child's behavior. By tracking, you can see your progress each week. At the end of this meeting, you'll leave with a plan to use incentives to increase the positive behaviors you've identified for your child. Before we begin with any new topics, do you have any questions about what we talked about during the last session?

Before we talk about your home practice, during the last session I asked you to think about messages from the past. Let's talk for a few minutes about this activity. What messages from the past did you think about during this week? What are the messages you have from your own parents, and what messages are you giving your child for the future?

For some families, this may be a very productive discussion. Many parents are blocked by past experiences with their own parents, and they benefit from processing past parenting and comparing the experience to their current experiences as a parent. This exercise may take more time with some families and should not be shortened.

Last week, you tracked your effective requests and your child's cooperation. You also tracked several pinpointed behaviors that you would like to see your child doing regularly, and you practiced praising cooperation. Let's talk about what you found out from tracking.

It is important to look at the tracking sheet if the parents bring it to the session. You can then talk through the information with respect to the following questions. If the parents have not brought in their tracking sheet, then you can gather information through the following questions. Again, reviewing the home practice validates its importance and your interest in their information. Ask:

➤ How did you pinpoint the behaviors?

➤ How many days of the week did you track?

➤ Were there certain steps that your child did more often?

➤ Did it seem to matter how you made a request in terms of your child's cooperation?

➤ Was there anything going on with your family that made tracking difficult?

➤ What did you learn about yourself or your child from this week's tracking?

Encourage both parents (if two parents are participating) to share their information.

BEHAVIOR-CHANGE PLANS

➤ Introduce use of incentives.

➤ Identify three types of incentives.

➤ Introduce incentive plans.

➤ Practice setting up a plan.

*The family management skill we're going to add this week is **incentives**, which means rewarding behavior we want to encourage. When we're reinforced for a behavior, we tend to repeat it. Many of us go to work each day because of the reinforcement of being paid. Some children choose to do homework because they are reinforced by the grades they are able to get. Other children might find hanging out with peers (to establish friendships) or playing computer games (to improve a previous score) more rewarding. Many young children are rewarded by simple praise and incentives, such as stickers.*

FAMILY MANAGEMENT SKILL: INCENTIVES

Incentives are a type of reinforcement. There are three features of incentives that make them work. We call this the PIE recipe:

*P: An incentive is experienced as **pleasant** to the child.*

*I: An incentive should occur **immediately** after a positive behavior is observed.*

*E: An incentive is given **every time** a youth engages in a positive behavior.*

Incentives should consistently follow behavior. "If you perform this behavior, then you'll earn this reward." When children haven't established a habit of performing a certain behavior or are having a hard time doing something, incentives can help encourage them. Providing incentives will help you see more of the behaviors you want your child to do. Pairing incentives with your praise and attention works best.

Many parents have concerns about rewarding children for behaviors they should be doing anyway. It is appropriate to process these feelings with parents and talk through the reasons why incentives are important to use in the home, even for behaviors a child should be doing.

When parents choose incentives that are meaningful to their children and provide them consistently, changes in behavior usually happen. Before we go further, let's talk about some common objections parents have when asked to use incentives to change their child's behavior.

Common complaints from parents about using incentives:

"A child shouldn't be rewarded for what she is supposed to be doing anyway."

Response: If your child is not doing what she is supposed to be doing, an incentive helps her get out of this pattern and back on the right track. Think of an incentive as a boost over a hurdle. Once she has learned to clear the hurdle, the incentive (boost) can get smaller and smaller.

"Incentives are bribes."

Response: No, not really. An incentive is encouragement and support. The most common incentives—praise and attention—simply feel good. Bribes are often related to carrying out negative behaviors. Also, bribes tend to be given before a behavior has been performed. Incentives follow good behavior. For example, if you give your child candy while you are on the phone to reduce whining, that is a bribe. If you give your child candy after you have hung up the phone to reward quiet behavior, that is an incentive.

"We don't have the resources in our family to provide incentives."

Response: Even when there is little money or few resources, incentives are available. Extra phone time or a later bedtime can be a powerful incentive and doesn't cost money. If resources are scarce, it may take longer for the child to earn the incentive. For example, if [Chris] wants a new sweater, she could earn a dollar or two toward the sweater for each week that she carries out her plan with her mom to keep her room clean. A young child can be rewarded with coupons that are made at home and cut out from paper.

"Rewarding children teaches them not to do things for their own enjoyment."

Response: Children do things they enjoy, like reading or other activities. Giving a reward for their efforts to do something that is hard for them or that they don't like won't change their enjoyment of other things. It will show them that you are trying to help them.

IDENTIFYING INCENTIVES

The first step in using incentives with your child is identifying things or activities that are affordable and enjoyable. There are three basic types of incentives:

- *Social incentives (praise)*

- *Activities (playing a game or cooking with a parent)*

- *Material incentives (money, food, treats)*

All three are effective.

You probably have a good idea of what would work for your [daughter]. If you aren't sure of what's currently reinforcing to your child, [she] can help you out when you set up the plan.

It's important that incentives are realistic and can be given on a daily basis.

Let's take a look at some commonly used incentives on Handout 3A.

Check five or six incentives that you would be willing to use and that you think would encourage your child. Try to select incentives from each category.

On Handout 3B, there's space to add your own ideas for incentives you think will encourage your child, including incentives you think you could provide daily and incentives that could be earned over time.

Discuss the list of incentives. Ask the parents what types of incentives they think will work with their child.

INCENTIVE PLANS

Now we're going to talk about incentive plans. These are simple written agreements between a parent and a child that specify what incentives *the child will earn for completing a set of pinpointed behaviors. It's still important to keep goals achievable so that you and your child don't become discouraged. Remember the three characteristics of achievable goals: **realistic**, **measurable**, and **under your control**.*

We suggest you start with a daily plan because it helps establish a routine. After your child has been successful with the daily plan, you can lengthen the time it takes to earn the incentive. Even if your child wants to work for a larger incentive, say renting a movie worth five tokens, [she] could earn a token each day toward the video.

Now let's take a look at Handout 3C, a plan that Chris's mom set up with her daughter. (Use Handout 3D for younger children.)

Go to Handout 3C (Handout 3D for young children)—the completed plan. Have parents decide on which days Chris earned an incentive. Draw attention to the goal of getting 4 out of 5 points to get an incentive. This is an important point to discuss. When we begin to make changes, we can't expect 100% all at once. So by going for about 80%, we are encouraging a good effort. This can change after a couple of weeks if children are successful.

Tip

Some parents may feel strongly that it is "all or nothing." If this is the case, explain the rationale for 80%, then go with what the parents want because this is their family. Usually, if you can suggest that the parent try 80% just for one week so that both the parent and the child can practice using an incentive plan, the parent will agree.

FAMILY COMMUNICATION SKILL: PROMPTING MOTIVATION IN YOUR CHILD AND ADOLESCENT

We recommend that you involve your child in developing the plan. Children always enjoy coming up with incentives. Once you have decided on the pinpointed behaviors to include in the plan, the most important thing to remember is to introduce the plan to your child by using a neutral request.

Setting up the plan with good communication skills doesn't guarantee cooperation, but it certainly can help promote it. Making effective requests and listening to your child's reactions will help you be successful and is a good way to teach your child the same skills.

Handout 3E includes a script you can use to practice setting up a plan with your child. By the way, this does not come naturally to most parents and takes lots of practice before it becomes a good habit.

DEVELOPMENTAL CONSIDERATIONS

It is essential to consider your child's developmental level when you set up incentives and plans. A younger child responds well to a sticker system or simple chart to earn basic rewards. As children develop, the plan may become more complicated and may involve adding up points and a range of incentives. It is important to develop a plan that is appropriate for your child's age and level.

For families with two parents:

Talk together and agree on the plan before you talk to your child. It's also a good idea to sit together when you discuss your plan. That shows you're in agreement and you're supporting one another. If you're a parent who is new to the family (for example, a new stepparent), it's often best to sit quietly and listen as the other parent presents the behavior-change request.

SETTING UP THE PLAN

Before you leave the meeting, you can fill out a sample plan using the pinpointed behaviors you tracked last week or make some changes in them based on our review. Then I'd like you to role-play setting up an incentive plan. It's helpful to practice what you'll say before actually talking with your child. I would like each of you to practice presenting and explaining the plan.

To help explain the plan, have different goals stated briefly on pieces of paper in a container for parents to select. For example, *doing chores around the house, homework, arguing,* or *coming home on time.* If parents select a goal that is one they actually have for their child, have them choose another one. Practice works best if it's not a real situation.

Therapists may role-play this activity with parents or have the two parents role-play it together. It is important for parents to practice these activities. Even though setting up a plan using an effective request may seem simple, it is much harder to use in our daily lives.

HOME PRACTICE

When you get home you can choose a time to work with your child on writing up the plan. You can fill out the sample on Handout 3F or 3G as a guide. I will give you a couple of extras to take home to work on with your child. It may be a good idea to wait until you get home and then ask for [her] help in coming up with the incentives. Handout 3H will offer guidance as you make the plan.

Parent Time

- ☐ Play a game for 15 minutes.
- ☐ Take a walk.
- ☐ Go out for ice cream.
- ☐ Work on a craft project for 15 minutes (e.g., woodworking, weaving, beading).
- ☐ Go to a park.
- ☐ Read a story to the child.

Activities

- ☐ Cook or bake together.
- ☐ Go to the movies.
- ☐ Have a night out (child's choice).
- ☐ Go fishing.
- ☐ Go hiking.
- ☐ Watch a video (just the two of you).
- ☐ Go to the park.

Home Resources

- ☐ Use the computer.
- ☐ Take bottles back to the store and keep or split the refund.
- ☐ Choose a special TV video game.
- ☐ Use parents' tools.

Privileges

- ☐ Choose a special TV program.
- ☐ Have a shared bedroom to him- or herself for one hour a day.
- ☐ Have first dibs on the bathroom in the morning (for specified amount of time).
- ☐ Get telephone time.
- ☐ Have permission to go to a special event (party, dance, concert).
- ☐ Have private time.
- ☐ Stay up a half hour later.
- ☐ Go swimming.
- ☐ Go out with friends.
- ☐ Have a friend over for the evening.
- ☐ Have a friend spend the night.
- ☐ Visit with grandparents, relatives.
- ☐ Look at a book in bed before lights out.
- ☐ Go to a friend's house.
- ☐ Have parent do one of the child's chores.

Incentives I can provide daily:

_____

_____

_____

_____

Incentives to be earned over time:

_____

_____

_____

_____

Goal: _clean room_   Week of: _November 16_

Responsibility	Sun.	Mon.	Tues.	Wed.	Thurs.	Fri.	Sat.
Clothes off the floor		✓	✓	✓		✓	✓
Bed made		✓					
Floor vacuumed		✓	✓			✓	✓
Desktop straightened		✓	✓			✓	
Laundry in hamper		✓	✓	✓		✓	
Total Daily Points	0	5	4	2	0	4	2

I, _____John_____, will earn a point for each of my responsibilities.

At the end of the day, if _____4_____ out of _____5_____ points have

been earned, I will receive an incentive from the list below.

_____John Jenks_____
Child's signature

I, _____John's mom_____, will check each day at ___6 p.m.___ to record _____John's_____

points. I will provide an incentive from the list below if _____he_____ earns the designated number

of points.

_____Monika Jenks_____
Parent's signature

Incentive List
30 minutes of video games
Having a friend over after school
Choice of dinner menu
Playing a game with Mom or Dad
One dollar

Goal: _brush teeth at night before bed_   Week of: _November 16_

Responsibility	Sun.	Mon.	Tues.	Wed.	Thurs.	Fri.	Sat.
Brush teeth at night before bed		✳	✧		✪	❖	✰

Note: For young children, use stickers on chart to indicate success.

I, _____Samara_____, will earn a sticker for each day that I _brush my teeth_.

At the end of the week, if _____5_____ out of _____7_____ stickers have

been earned, I will receive an incentive from the list below.

_____Samara_____
Child's signature

I, _Samara's mom_, will check each day at _6 p.m._ to record _Samara's_

points. I will provide an incentive from the list below if _____she_____ earns the designated number

of points.

_____Amy Webster_____
Parent's signature

Incentive List
Story time with Mom or Dad
Having a friend over after school
Going to the park
Playing a game with Mom or Dad
Ice cream treat

From *Everyday Parenting: A Professional's Guide to Building Family Management Skills*, © 2012 by T. J. Dishion, E. A. Stormshak, and K. A. Kavanagh, Champaign, IL: Research Press (www.researchpress.com, 800-519-2707).

What to Say

- "I/we want to talk to you about the problem of _____."

- "Because it is important to me/us that you do this, I/we have broken the plan down into some simple steps."

- "Each step is worth points. I/we will keep track of how you do each day, and each day that you earn _____ points, you will earn an incentive."

- "Now, I'd/we'd like to hear your ideas for things you could earn."

- "Do you have any questions? Is everything clear?"

- "I/we hope you earn lots of incentives!"

From *Everyday Parenting: A Professional's Guide to Building Family Management Skills,* © 2012 by T. J. Dishion, E. A. Stormshak, and K. A. Kavanagh, Champaign, IL: Research Press (www.researchpress.com, 800-519-2707).

Goal: _____ Week of: _____

Responsibility	Sun.	Mon.	Tues.	Wed.	Thurs.	Fri.	Sat.
Total Daily Points							

I, _____, will earn a point for each of my responsibilities.

At the end of the day, if _____ out of _____ points have

been earned, I will receive an incentive from the list below.

_____

Child's signature

I, _____, will check each day at _____ to record _____

points. I will provide an incentive from the list below if _____ earns the designated number

of points.

_____

Parent's signature

Incentive List
30 minutes of video games
Having a friend over after school
Choice of dinner menu
Playing a game with Mom or Dad
One dollar

Goal: _____ Week of: _____

Responsibility	Sun.	Mon.	Tues.	Wed.	Thurs.	Fri.	Sat.

Note: For young children, use stickers on chart to indicate success.

I, _____, will earn a sticker for each day that I _____.

At the end of the week, if _____ out of _____ stickers have

been earned, I will receive an incentive from the list below.

_____
Child's signature

I, _____, will check each day at _____ to record _____

points. I will provide an incentive from the list below if _____ earns the designated number

of points.

_____
Parent's signature

Incentive List
Story time with Mom or Dad
Having a friend over after school
Going to the park
Playing a game with Mom or Dad
Ice cream treat

Have I talked with my child and explained what each of us will do?   ☐ Yes ☐ No

Have I chosen behaviors that my child is capable of doing and that are   ☐ Yes ☐ No
realistic, measurable, specific, and under my control?

Have I broken the behaviors into small-enough steps?   ☐ Yes ☐ No

Have my child and I come up with an incentive or list of incentives?   ☐ Yes ☐ No

Have I specified a time to check the behavior each day?   ☐ Yes ☐ No

Is the plan appropriate for my child's developmental level?   ☐ Yes ☐ No

Behavior-Change Plans

Reviewing, Revising, and Reducing Barriers to Change

OVERVIEW AND RATIONALE

The best way to appreciate a family dynamic is to try to change it. Lessons are always learned about a parent and a family following an attempt to implement a behavior-change plan. A successful effort will go a long way toward motivating parents to continue to maintain family management practices. A failed effort can be demoralizing to a parent and lead to disengagement in the change process or, worse, to blaming the child or adolescent for making change difficult. For this reason, we think of home practice as experiments: something is learned from both success and failure. The important feature of a home-practice experiment is learning from the experience. In this session, we support parents in their effort to review and revise their behavior-change plans and to assess their own thoughts and feelings about behavior change. A better understanding of themselves as parents will help reduce personal barriers to parents' positive behavior support and make positive changes in their family.

There are at least four ways in which a behavior-change plan can be unsuccessful. In one, the behavior-change plan is undermined by the parent–child interaction dynamic. For example, if a parent tends to avoid interactions with his or her child or is distracted from parenting, there may be little discussion of the point chart, and the child therefore loses interest. Alternatively, a parent may be emotionally overengaged and may blame or criticize a child on days that are less successful, emphasizing the negative over the positive. A child or adolescent, understandably, would prefer that there not be a behavior-change plan. The interaction pattern undermines the goal of positive family change. We suggest that the parent briefly review the behavior-change plan daily if possible. Role-playing with the parent a constructive approach to reviewing the behavior-change plan may also be helpful for some families. Second, as discussed in Session 3, a parent's life may be overly busy or chaotic, and for this reason the parent is unable to be consistent. If this is the case and the parent is ambivalent about changing his or her own life to prioritize parenting, then it would be helpful to have a motivational discussion about this topic. ("What are the advantages to you and your family of working 70 hours a week?" "What are the advantages to you and your family of working on this behavior-change plan every day?" "What are the costs of each?") This kind of discussion helps lead parents to consider their own motivations and, perhaps, to live a family life more consistent with their own values.

The third major problem is that a child can lose interest even when the parent is consistent, reviews the behavior-change plan, and keeps a positive focus. There are a few possible reasons for children losing interest. One is that they already get so many rewarding experiences that are "freebies" that the incentives of the behavior-change plan are simply less valuable. If this is the case, it suggests that the parents need to reevaluate their child's or adolescent's overall level of rewarding experiences, especially in light of the problem behavior. It will be necessary to reevaluate the incentives and ensure that those offered for a successful day or week are really of interest to the youth and, perhaps, to make some of the freebies contingent. This can be problematic if the child lives in two households, with one household being entirely noncontingent. The second reason a youth may lose interest is that the incentives simply are not interesting to him or her. This is easy to resolve by asking the child to offer suggestions, then revising the incentive plan.

Another reason for a child's losing interest may be that the parent takes incentives away when there has been a problem behavior that is not on the chart, even though the child followed through with the positive behaviors for that day. For example, the focus is on chores, but the parent gets upset at the child for swearing at her brother and calling him an unthinkable name. The upset parent withdraws the reward earned that day. It is human to want to do this, but it is counterproductive for the behavior-change plan. Each problem behavior should be dealt with separately and should not disrupt parents' efforts to teach new behaviors.

Fourth, sometimes a parent's thoughts and feelings are barriers to positive family change. Several third-generation cognitive-behavioral therapies address this issue, such as dialectical behavior therapy and acceptance and commitment therapy. In all approaches, the first step in making progress is to identify the thoughts or feelings that might interfere with implementing a behavior-change plan. The second step is for the parent to become more mindful of those thoughts and feelings daily and to notice when they come up and how they interfere. Acknowledge that it is okay for parents to have those thoughts and feelings and to be consistent with the behavior-change plan despite them. So parents must learn to be positive and consistent in a behavior-change plan, even though they may be concerned that it will upset the delicate balance of a parent–child relationship. Alternatively, the parent may have doubts that she or he can make these changes successfully. The final exercise in this session is a self-assessment of thoughts and feelings about change and a home exercise in which we ask the parent to track these thoughts and feelings daily.

SUGGESTED TOOLS

➤ Videotaped examples of parents reviewing a point chart or behavior-change plan that is developmentally appropriate for the targeted child

➤ Handout for parent self-assessment

➤ Behavior-change plan forms that are developmentally appropriate for the child or adolescent and are tailored to the child and family

➤ Whiteboard, chalkboard, or large sheets of paper

SESSION OBJECTIVES

➤ Role-play with parents their approach to reviewing the behavior-change plan.

➤ Support the parents' skills at revising behavior-change plans if the plans are initially unsuccessful.

➤ Help parents identify their thought-and-feeling barriers to implementing a behavior-change plan and providing contingent incentives.

➤ Set parents up for a successful behavior-change plan experiment for the next week.

COMMON PITFALLS AND SOLUTIONS

Motivation

A well-developed behavior change plan may not work because the caregiver is unable to be involved, enthusiastic, and consistent on a daily basis. Children of any age will lose interest quickly if the parent is not attentive about the plan. Parents may be resistant to the plan or unmotivated about executing it because of time constraints, stress level, or inability to regulate their own emotions so that they are consistent day to day. One way to get the ball rolling is to take responsibility when the behavior change plan doesn't work ("I should have considered doing this in the morning rather than in the evening"). Another is to simplify the plan so it is more likely to be used consistently. A plan that is delivered consistently for one hour each day is better than one with a daylong strategy that is executed inconsistently. With respect to parents' motivation to change and engage in treatment, a very limited but consistent behavior-change plan is far better than an ambitious, unsuccessful plan.

Tailoring

It is common for parents to create an initial plan for a child that does not work the first time and needs to be adapted over several sessions. Many factors may affect the success of the plan, including the child's developmental level and the choice of incentives for the child. Make sure that parents stay aware that behavior-change plans take time to develop and to adapt for each child. Then, when the plan fails, parents will not feel discouraged as they tailor and change the plan accordingly. Consider the example from Session 3 in which the therapist cut and pasted the child's photograph on a dollar bill and created "Jacob bucks." It may be that this incentive was interesting to Jacob for only a few days, and then he lost interest in earning the bucks. The plan should then be tailored to include a wider range of incentives for Jacob.

Structuring Sessions to Reduce Barriers

This session will depend on the specifics of the success and failure of the behavior-change plan. The therapist's questions should be diagnostic of how to revise the plan and of what aspect of this session is most relevant to this particular family. Parents may be resistant to this session if they simply did not put their behavior-change plan into action, so it will be prudent for the therapist to use motivational strategies to help the parents identify their own priorities with respect to this plan. Reviewing the parents' own issues (e.g., stress, depression) as possible limits to setting the plan into action may also be helpful.

SETTING THE AGENDA

Good to see you again. Last week you started the behavior-change plan [or point/sticker chart] for [Chris]. Today I'd like to spend quite a bit of time with you going over that experience and troubleshooting any problems that came up. Before we begin, has anything happened since the last time we met that I should know about before we move forward?

If anything has happened that would affect parents' skill development during the session, it should be briefly addressed, and they should be asked if they are ready to continue the work started in the previous session.

I have planned that we would cover the following today (write on a piece of paper, whiteboard, etc., so the parents can see the list):

- Review behavior-change plan, troubleshoot problems.

- Practice reviewing the plan with your child or teenager.

- Revise the behavior-change plan for the future.

- Do exercise on parent self-statements.

- Discuss the home practice experiments.

Does this seem doable for today? Is there anything else you would like to address?

Be responsive to the parents' concerns, or tailor the list by adding items such as *two parents using praise* if you want to deal with a family dynamic in which only one parent acknowledges a child's behavior and you feel this could change.

REVIEW OF SESSION 3

During the last session we talked about positive reinforcement and behavior plans as our family management skills. Setting up an incentive plan with your child was the communication skill we worked on and that you practiced this week. Do you have any questions about what we talked about last week?

REVIEW OF HOME PRACTICE

The home practice for the last session was to set up a plan with your child, keep track of the pinpointed behaviors, and give your child an incentive when [she] made at least 80% of [her] points. Let's review how your week went.

Ask the parents about their plan with their child. For focus, use review questions to avoid interrogating parents. If the family didn't develop the plan, they can answer the question about what interfered with getting it started:

➤ Were you able to set up the plan?

➤ Was it helpful to role-play explaining the plan to your child?

➤ How did your child react to the plan?

➤ Did your child help decide on incentives?

➤ How many days did you review the plan?

➤ How many days did your child earn an incentive?

➤ If you were able to set up a plan, what supported getting that done?

➤ If you did not set up a plan, what interfered with getting the plan going?

Frame parents' answers to the last two questions in terms of whether a person or an outside influence interfered with their ability to carry out their goals. Possible problems might include parents' work schedules, parent or child illness, unexpected events, parent fatigue, child's resistance to activity, and parent discouragement from being unable to track each day.

Factors supporting success might include tracking at the same time each day, receiving reminders from child and partner, refusing to make negative self-statements when tracking wasn't done, not planning other activities during the time set aside to track, and selecting alternative incentives when they were too stressed or short of time. Discussing support and interference in this way can help parents identify why they were not successful and how to work around interference during the next week.

Just by reviewing this home practice, it reminds us of what's involved in making a change in a child's behavior.

It's typical for some plans to work smoothly and others not. This should be stated and normalized.

FAMILY MANAGEMENT SKILL: REVIEW, REVISE, AND REDUCE BARRIERS TO CHANGE

This week, our family management skill continues to be positive behavior support. Today we will focus on how best to review a behavior-change plan, strategies for revising one that is not working, and ways to reduce barriers to effective behavior-change plans.

We'll also focus on things you can do to help plans work better. Even if you had a good week or have successfully used a plan in the past, it's likely there are things you can do to help maintain the plan longer and make it more a part of your family routine.

We briefly discussed some of these things at our last meeting. Here are six questions to answer as you either set up or continue to use your incentive plan. When you can answer yes to these questions, you are on your way to making a plan that will work.

Questions for Parents to Ask

➤ Have I talked with my child and explained what each of us will do?

➤ Have I chosen behaviors that are realistic, measurable/specific, and under my control that my child is capable of doing?

➤ Have I broken the behaviors into small enough steps?

➤ Have my child and I come up with an incentive or list of incentives?

➤ Have I specified a time to check the behavior each day?

➤ Is the plan appropriate for the child's developmental level?

Things to Remember When Reviewing a Behavior Plan

➤ Review the plan each day.

➤ Check each step of the plan.

➤ Praise positive behaviors.

➤ Give incentives immediately after they are earned.

Things to Avoid When Reviewing a Plan

➤ Reviewing the plan if you are upset (Come back in about 30 minutes and try again, or ask your partner to review it.)

➤ Taking away an incentive the child has earned (When children misbehave, parents can be tempted to withhold incentives even if the child has fulfilled the plan. Positive and negative behavior are separate and should be responded to separately.)

➤ Blaming

➤ Lecturing

On Handout 4A, you'll find some common situations that occur when parents begin using incentive plans. Let's read through these situations so you can be prepared if they come up for you.

FAMILY COMMUNICATION SKILL: SELF-STATEMENTS

➤ Introduce the concept of negative and positive self-statements.

➤ Have parents identify self-statements about change.

Obstacles

As parents, you know that your best intentions aren't always realized. Because of daily activities and problems (for example, hectic schedules), it's hard to be consistent. We call events that interfere with parent goals **obstacles***.*

A common obstacle is parents not believing that they can change their child's behavior. Negative self-statements, such as "She never listens to me," can make you feel ineffective and reduce your motivation to make necessary changes. Positive self-statements, such as "I really think my child can change," encourage you to continue your efforts.

Assessing your beliefs is an important part of changing behavior and something we seldom make time for. For the next few minutes, complete the Parent in the Mirror exercise on Handout 4B.

This task may be difficult for some parents. It is common for parents with children who have behavior problems to feel negative about their children. Therapists should take time with this task if needed.

Let's hear some of the positive and negative self-statements you wrote. Often the hardest ones to come up with are the positive self-statements. What did you write?

Negative self-statements about your ability to make changes may be a result of a lack of support. What you want to change in your child's behavior is often not something [she] wants to change. For example, your [daughter] may think [she] shouldn't have to do chores or homework or cooperate with your requests. Making family changes requires support, and parents can't depend on children for this support. Parents need to get support from other adults. Who are supportive adults in your life who can help you make changes in your parenting?

With parents, talk about who is supportive in their lives and how these people might provide even better support. Unfortunately, some parents may not be able to identify any supportive adults. These parents should be encouraged to think of parents of their child's friends whom they respect or perhaps older adults who have raised their children successfully whom they could begin using as supports.

Barriers to doing this task should be discussed and role-played.

HOME PRACTICE

Handout 3F has a behavior plan form for adolescents, and Handout 3G has a plan for younger children. Briefly review how to fill out the plan for parents who need a refresher. Help parents troubleshoot any problems from the previous weeks in relation to their tracking.

> *This time you'll continue to use the incentive plan form, found on Handouts 3F and 3G. If the plan you used last session is working well, stick with it for another week. If you didn't set one up or if there were some obstacles, start again. Remember, start with a neutral request, involve your child in the choice of incentives, and review the plan daily.*

> *I'd also like to follow up on what we talked about during this meeting and have you write down any self-statements you make this week about your child's ability to change and your ability to help [her] change. There's a form for this purpose on Handout 4C. It's normal to have some thoughts that aren't positive, but you'll notice that as your child's behavior improves, so will your positive self-statements about [her] and about your abilities.*

"My schedule is too full to review the plan each day—should I still try to do a behavior plan?"

The goal of the plan is to teach your child positive behaviors by encouraging daily efforts. Ideally, a plan should be reviewed daily, but sometimes family schedules may not allow for that. If you can't check the plan every day, check it as often as you can.

"My child isn't interested in the plan, and we seem to battle over getting it done."

There could be several reasons why your child isn't interested in the plan. First, check to make sure the task isn't too difficult and that it is clearly specified. Are you reviewing progress and offering praise for what your child has done each day? Your interest and words of encouragement for efforts can go a long way. ("Good, you got all the dishes to the sink and scraped the plates. Maybe tomorrow you will remember to do the other parts of the chore so I can give you your reward.")

Your child may already be getting many incentives without cooperating with the plan. If so, you'll want to change what your child gets as a "freebie" and what he or she earns as an incentive. Another situation might be that your child is doing many things that are positive without being reinforced. It might be useful to put one or two of these behaviors on the plan. In that way, you are more likely to be able to focus on something positive.

You may want to offer extra points for doing the pinpointed behaviors without a reminder from you. For example, if each step is worth two points, increase the value to four points if it's done without a reminder, then adjust the number needed to earn the incentive.

"After a few weeks, my child is no longer interested in the plan, and the behavior is already better."

Don't give up. If the behavior is what you want it to be, tell your child that you are proud of his or her accomplishments. At this point, you might want to consider renegotiating the plan to:

- Reinforce your child for carrying out the goal without reminders.

- Ask for more successful days of the behavior to get the same incentives.

- Select new incentives.

Another option is to use the plan for another skill or behavior you want your child to achieve. Just remember—behavior plans provide a boost and help kids get back on track doing what you want them to do on a regular basis. They also help you stay consistent in your expectations and in your recognition of positive behaviors.

*Put an **N** next to the beliefs that are negative self-statements about change and a **P** next to those that are positive.*

_____ 1. "He'll never change. He's just like his uncle."

_____ 2. "Before I deal with Michael's negative attitude, I need a better idea of what the problem is."

_____ 3. "Next week, I'll try offering Alison the incentive of extra phone time for doing at least 30 minutes of homework a day."

_____ 4. "There's something wrong with her head—I've never understood why she behaves like this."

_____ 5. "I've tried using incentives before and they don't work with John."

_____ 6. "Things always get in the way of us solving this problem—nothing will ever change."

_____ 7. "My husband and I need to talk about a way to make time to track Maria's chores every day."

_____ 8. "If I take one step at a time and stick to my goals, I can make a difference."

_____ 9. "A program like this will not work with a kid like Sarah."

_____ 10. "I'll talk to the group leader about Karim to see if there is anything we should do differently."

Positive self-statements I make about my ability to influence my child's behavior:

_____

_____

Negative self-statements I make about my ability to influence my child's behavior:

_____

_____

From *Everyday Parenting: A Professional's Guide to Building Family Management Skills,* © 2012 by T. J. Dishion, E. A. Stormshak, and K. A. Kavanagh, Champaign, IL: Research Press (www.researchpress.com, 800-519-2707).

Write any self-statements you think or say aloud about your child or yourself this week.

1. _____

2. _____

3. _____

4. _____

5. _____

6. _____

7. _____

8. _____

9. _____

10. _____

Monitoring Daily Activities

Daily Structure and Listening

OVERVIEW AND RATIONALE

The foundation of healthy limit setting is monitoring children's and adolescents' daily activities. When children enter school, they begin spending more time with peers than with parents. In today's world, some children run the risk of being highly influenced by peers when parents are uninvolved, not attending to parenting, or simply unaware of children's daily activities.

Parental monitoring is a two-way street. Some children, and especially adolescents, are challenging to monitor. When youths become involved in problem behavior, they actively avoid adult supervision and tracking and therefore require more effort, attention, and skill to monitor than most children. In this session, four aspects (the four Cs) of parental monitoring—clear rules, consistency, checking up, and communication—are described, and parents are invited to use the four Cs to set up a daily structure for their child or adolescent.

Listening skills are a fundamental aspect of parental monitoring of daily activities. Careful and skillful listening opens a window into the lives of children and adolescents when they are away from the family, experiencing the world, potentially in danger of getting into trouble, or simply unsafe. There are several ways in which parents can unintentionally turn off communication with their child. First, they may seem uninterested in the life of the child, and it shows when the child talks. This can happen because of distractions in the parents' lives, such as stressful work situations, divorce or marital conflict, or other personal troubles. Second, parents can cut off communication by reacting emotionally to what their children say or do so that the children learn to avoid talking about their lives. Being critical of a youngster is a third sure way to stop the flow of communication.

Listening skills are vital to all close relationships. Actively listening to what someone is saying can make the difference between having a rich conversation or one that seems to fall flat. In this session, active listening skills are introduced and role-plays are structured. Developing listening skills requires practice because habitual patterns of communication often disrupt the interaction of speaking and listening.

Parental monitoring also requires communication with other adults. Most often, this involves getting to know the parents of the children a child spends time with. For children with trouble in school, effective monitoring is critical to promoting a student's progress in behavior and academic skills. In this session, both skills—active listening and effective monitoring—are discussed, and role-plays are suggested. These skills are especially useful if a parent has a style that would lead to unproductive interactions with other parents or teachers—interactions that are not in the child's best interest.

Monitoring a high-risk youth requires cooperation among parents. Families defined by two homes (divorced, joint custody), estranged marital partners, or two parents with very different parenting styles can disrupt monitoring. In situations such as these, success in improving parental monitoring is diminished if adults do not "agree to agree." Thus the four Cs of monitoring serve as a foundation for promoting structure in a youth's life, and an intervention with multiple adults may be required to get them all "on the same page." Two parents with different styles may need to become more aware of their differences and reach a compromise. Such families often develop elaborate and highly stable patterns, with one parent being strict and the other parent being more lenient and forgiving, undoing the efforts of the parent who is strict. This pattern, if left unchanged, can escalate so that each parent's style is exaggerated to a point that is detrimental to the youth, who may inadvertently play one parent against the other. The exercises in this session can address this pattern.

SUGGESTED TOOLS

➤ Videotape on parental monitoring (the four Cs) and/or parental listening

➤ Videotape of parent talking with teacher

➤ Handout on the four Cs of parental monitoring

➤ Worksheet on rules that structure the daily activities of youths

➤ Whiteboard, chalkboard, or large sheets of paper

SESSION OBJECTIVES

➤ Role-play talking to parents or teachers to open communication that facilitates structuring and monitoring youth activities.

➤ Role-play active listening skills with parents.

➤ Discuss with parents how to practice at home generating rules and guidelines that provide a daily structure to enhance parental monitoring.

COMMON PITFALLS AND SOLUTIONS

Motivation

Motivation is a significant component of both listening and monitoring. It is not uncommon to observe parent–youth interactions that may seem problematic. For example, when a 14-year-old youth tells a story about a time he was out all night unsupervised with friends and the parent appears to be unconcerned, we refer to this style as the *sibling parent*. This parenting style requires a motivational discussion about the pros and cons of parental monitoring, with some very clear information given to the parent about the risk associated with deviant peer exposure and the like. Two common myths about monitoring young adolescents are that (1) older children can be responsible for their own behavior and (2) monitoring an adolescent implies that the parent doesn't trust him or her. Both of these myths can be discussed with a focus on safety, in that the risks to safety are actually higher in adolescence and that parents need to attend to the details. Trust grows from better communication and monitoring. We recommend that the motivational issue be addressed before proceeding to support the parent in developing his or her skills.

Tailoring

Tailoring in this session essentially establishes the foundation for more work on setting limits. The exercise What Kind of Parent Are You? helps establish a collaborative relationship with parents about their collective strengths and weaknesses in setting limits in general and in parental monitoring in particular. For parents who have strong limit-setting skills but are in disrupted family circumstances, such as marital conflict or postdivorce communication patterns, all that may be required is an agreement about rules that are consistent across the two households. On the other hand, for sibling parents, the concept of parent-generated rules may provoke anxiety, and if this is the case, it is helpful to discuss the parents' emotions about establishing rules and functioning as leaders in the family. Loss of a relationship with their child is a common concern that underlies parents' reluctance to set limits. This concern should be validated, and information should be provided about how providing structure and protecting children strengthen relationships in the long term. Finally, the parental networking and school communication part of this session may be less relevant for some parents than for others. However, most parents of adolescents will be able to identify a peer of their child's whose parents they would like to know better.

Structuring Sessions to Reduce Barriers

Data from the Family Check-Up are used to structure this session. These data offer clear insight into parents' strengths and weaknesses in limit setting. The feedback session likely resulted in a collaborative relationship with the parents on areas of focus for limit setting. It is important to be active in this session, to have fun with the role-plays on parental networking, and to avoid letting parents get into blaming traps, such as "I don't have a problem at my house, but his mom doesn't set limits." Stay focused on the here and now and what you are potentially able to do with the parent in the room.

SETTING THE AGENDA

Good to see you again. As we agreed, I plan to work with you on looking at the structure you have in place for [Chris] and to talk about "tricks of the trade" that might be useful for you in monitoring and supervising. Before we begin, has anything happened since the last time we met that I should know about?

If anything has happened that would affect parents' skill development during the session, it should be briefly addressed, and they should be asked if they are ready to continue the work started in the previous session.

I have planned that we would cover the following today (write on a piece of paper, whiteboard, etc., so the parents can see the list):

- Review any past work with the parents.

- Discuss the four Cs of parental monitoring.

- Discuss listening skills with children and adolescents.

- Do the exercise What Kind of Parent Are You?

- Discuss the home practice experiments.

Does this seem doable for today? Is there anything else you would like to address today?

REVIEW OF SESSION 4

If you have previously worked with parents on a behavior-change plan, you will, of course, review how that is going and see if they would like to make any adjustments.

Last week, we talked about behavior-change plans, and we went over the plan you are using with [Chris] to reduce [the level of arguments]. Let's review the plan now for a few minutes. How is the plan going? How have the revisions to the plan worked out? How is your child responding to the plan?

If this is your first meeting since the Family Check-Up or after a long period of time, this opening question may lead to responses about events that significantly change the nature of your work with a family. At some point, you would acknowledge that a lot is happening and defer the content of this session to the next time you meet to be empathic to the parents' situation and to maximize their ability to work on their parenting skills.

FAMILY MANAGEMENT SKILL: MONITORING

During this meeting, we will talk about a set of important skills that can all be grouped under the term **monitoring**. *As you know, good monitoring skills help you:*

- *Know what your child is doing*

- *Set limits*

- *Offer guidance in problem situations*

Monitoring is the key to effective parenting during both early childhood and the teenage years. It is especially important as your child gains more independence and increasingly spends time away from home. In this meeting, we'll talk about some aspects of monitoring that help you meet this challenging period.

We have identified the four Cs of monitoring, and they are listed on Handout 5A.

NETWORKING WITH OTHER PARENTS

Introduce the following format for parental networking.

For younger children, it is important for parents to network with other parents at school to provide social opportunities, such as play dates for your child. Having a community of parents at your child's school will also give you information about your child's behavior, your child's social skills, and community events and activities. Social interaction outside of school is critical to your child's development of good social skills.

Knowing the parents of your child's friends helps you supervise your child. Have you called or introduced yourself to the parents of your child's friends? Was that a positive experience? If you haven't, I encourage you to do so. If you need some help, try using the example on Handout 5B as a starting place.

EXERCISE: WHAT KIND OF PARENT ARE YOU?

Now we're going to turn to the second family management skill of this meeting, **limit setting**.

Sometimes it's easier to see what we are doing when we can step back and read about other parents.

Is there a family like yours when it comes to setting limits? As we read through each parent description on the second page of Handout 5C, you can see if there is one that seems like you. Or maybe your style is a combination of descriptions. Also, think about the way you set limits, along with a strength and an area for improvement in your limit setting. I'll check in with you as we go along.

FAMILY COMMUNICATION SKILL: ACTIVE LISTENING

*Active listening is a set of communication skills to use when your child is talking. Active listening means that you are making an effort to understand what your child is really saying. Too often, we interrupt, give advice, or get angry when our children tell us what is going on in their lives. Active listening is a way to get information. The active listening skills we will learn in this session are **encouraging** and **paraphrasing**.*

Active Listening Skills

Encouraging: The purpose of encouraging is to show interest in what is being said and to keep your child talking. There are three main points to remember when you are encouraging your child to share information. If you already do these things, then this will be a reminder of what you're doing that encourages your child to talk to you.

- *Look at your child.*

- *Nod your head yes or say uh-huh in a positive or neutral tone when the child pauses.*

- *Don't say anything else.*

Ask parents what happens in their home when their child tries to tell them something they do not like hearing about, such as a friend being kicked out of school, a friend being arrested for carrying a weapon, or that there are drugs at school.

Paraphrasing: This is another simple, active listening skill to use when your child is talking. All you do is repeat what your child has said to you. This shows that you understand the facts and that you're listening, avoiding one of the most common complaints, "You never listen to me!"

We're going to practice active listening skills today before trying them at home.

If you are working with two parents, they can enact these role-plays with your coaching. If you are working with one parent, put yourself in the parent role first to demonstrate the skills.

Active Listening Practice

Finish the scenarios with one parent role-playing the child and the other parent or leader role-playing the parent. The "child" should begin by trying to relate the story. First, the "parent" should role-play the wrong way of listening to the child so that the conversation stops and the "parent" doesn't get all the information. Next, the "parent" should use active listening skills to find out about the "child's" good and bad decisions.

Leshawndra

Background: Leshawndra has been getting into trouble at school, mostly in her relationships with peers. The teacher reports that she is aggressive at times, uses name calling, and often provokes conflicts and disagreements. Based on Leshawndra's reports at home, Leshawndra's mom feels like the school is not sensitive to her daughter and that it is her classmates who are causing the problem.

Story: Leshawndra pulled a girl's hair in the lunch line today, and the girl's two friends came over and pushed Leshawndra and told her to leave their friend alone. The duty personnel observed the situation, stopped the conflict, and moved Leshawndra to the back of the line.

Scene: Leshawndra's mom picks her up from school and sees that Leshawndra is upset. "What happened at school today? You look upset."

Leshawndra: "I got put in the back of the line just because Tosha and Melanie were picking on me!"

Alberto

Background: Alberto's parents do not want him to spend time with some neighborhood peers who live about a block away. Alberto's best friend, Pete, has an older brother who is involved in this group. Pete's older brother is in eighth grade, and Pete and Alberto are in third grade.

Story: This afternoon, while Alberto's dad was getting his car fixed, Alberto and Pete went to Pete's house to pick up his soccer ball and ran into the guys, who were smoking and sitting around talking and laughing. They were very friendly with the boys and offered them a cigarette, which they both refused.

Scene: After about an hour, Alberto leaves and is going home, and his dad pulls up and picks him up in the car.

Dad: "Hey, son, what have you been doing?"

Alberto: "I was just walking home from Pete's. We were going to get his soccer ball ..."

Katy

Background: Katy is an early-maturing girl whose parents are concerned about her involvement with boys.

Story: Today a boy who has been calling Katy at home put his arm around her when they were walking down the hall at school. She asked him politely to take it off, but he acted as if she were joking. The principal happened to see them and called them into her office to talk about showing affection at school. Katy later asked the boy not to call her anymore and told him she never wanted to see him again.

Scene: Katy is riding with her mother and seems upset. Mom asks what happened at school today.

Katy: "The principal called me into her office."

Elicit responses. Let the parent know that active listening skills allow children to express their feelings and opinions without interruption and that it feels good to them knowing someone's really listening.

HOME PRACTICE

Next time your child starts to talk with you, try these active listening skills—you'll be surprised what your kids will tell you if you don't interrupt, get angry, or give advice. You can complete a form on Handout 5D after you do the activity with your child this week.

I would like you to call the parents of one of your child's friends. If you have done this a lot, then follow what you normally do. If this is something new, try following the sample provided on Handout 5B.

There is also a limit-setting assessment on Handout 5E I'd like you to fill out. It will help you prepare for the work we will do next session.

Clear Rules

Have only a few clear rules about your child's activities. Some good examples include providing phone numbers of places where he or she will be, giving you 24-hour notice for a party or staying overnight, not having friends over when parents aren't home, and no hitting his or her sibling.

Consistency

Each time a rule is followed, give praise.

Checking Up

Every now and then, let your child know that you made the rule because you care about her and her safety. Check to see that your child is at the number or location she gave you. Checking up also helps teach your child accountability and to take your rules seriously.

Communication

Communicating with other parents and school staff in advance about your son or daughter will give you an advantage if a problem develops. Other parents can also be a powerful resource for information about your child. Some of you already may have a communication procedure with your school, such as a home–school card, that gives you weekly or daily information.

How to Get Started

"Hi, this is Tracy's mom. Do you have a couple of minutes? I want to introduce myself and share some information about our family since our kids are spending so much time together."

What to Share

Share family information and some of your rules, such as:

- "Emma can't be out past nine o'clock."

- "I also wanted to share our work schedules so you'll know when we're home."

- "Would you feel comfortable sharing a little about your family and some rules you have for Kristen so that I can support those rules when she's in my home?"

*Which parent category or combination of parent categories are most like you? (Parent descriptions are on **next** page.)*

_____

It's possible that none of these parents describes you. What is your story?

_____

_____

_____

What is one strength that you bring to setting limits with children?

_____

In what area would you like to improve?

_____

_____

From *Everyday Parenting: A Professional's Guide to Building Family Management Skills,* © 2012 by T. J. Dishion, E. A. Stormshak, and K. A. Kavanagh, Champaign, IL: Research Press (www.researchpress.com, 800-519-2707).

What Kind of Parent Are You?

The Parent–Friend

Donna has been a single parent for about 2 years. She and her daughter, Caitlyn, became close after the divorce. There was no secret they did not share, including all the trauma of the breakup. Caitlyn is now 12 years old and has started spending time with older friends, including some boys. She is not coming home on time, nor does she let Donna know where she is. Because she and Caitlyn have been so close, Donna is having trouble setting limits with her daughter and giving her consequences.

The Parent–Boss

When Jim was a child, his parents were pretty strict and let him know when he broke the rules. He always "paid for it." There was also a lot of yelling when he got into trouble. Now when his own kids irritate him or break the rules, he quickly becomes angry, sometimes coming down too heavily or being too quick to give a consequence. Later, he's often sorry because his relationships with his son and daughter suffer. He's been told that it would be a good idea to "loosen up" on his kids. He agrees, but it doesn't come naturally.

Parents at War

Tomas and Maria have different parenting styles. Maria is strict and Tomas is easygoing. They haven't learned how to work as a team and blend their two styles. Because they don't always agree, they sometimes do things that weaken each other. For example, Tomas will say it's okay to do something that Maria has said no to, or Maria will step in when Tomas is dealing with the kids, making him look and feel ineffective. The kids tend to use their parents' differences to their own advantage.

The Unavailable Parent

Dave is a single father. He has three children ranging in age from 5 to 15. Dave goes to school during the day and works on weekends, as well as several evenings each week. The oldest child, Sherry, takes care of the other kids when Dave isn't at home. Often, when Dave gets home, Sherry complains that the other kids won't follow the rules. When Sherry complains, Dave gets frustrated, withdraws, and goes to bed for some much-needed rest.

Parent/Stepparent

Karen and Sam recently married. Karen has two sons (7 and 9), and Sam has one daughter (12). They all live together. Karen's sons accept the limits Karen sets, but they argue and do not observe the limits Sam sets. Sam and Karen often argue about this situation. For the past couple of months, Sam has been unsure of what role to take when setting limits with the boys. He is aware that certain limits must be set, even if Karen is not at home, but he hesitates in order to avoid a fight.

From *Everyday Parenting: A Professional's Guide to Building Family Management Skills,* © 2012 by T. J. Dishion, E. A. Stormshak, and K. A. Kavanagh, Champaign, IL: Research Press (www.researchpress.com, 800-519-2707).

Did you …

Look at your child?	☐ Yes	☐ No
Show understanding?	☐ Yes	☐ No
Nod your head or say uh-huh?	☐ Yes	☐ No
Practice patience?	☐ Yes	☐ No
Summarize what your child said?	☐ Yes	☐ No
Emphasize positive behaviors?	☐ Yes	☐ No

What was your child's mood?   ☐ Positive   ☐ Neutral   ☐ Negative

What specific things did you learn from your child?

_____

_____

_____

What is the hardest part of setting limits with your child?

_____

_____

_____

_____

What strategies have you used to address this problem?

_____

_____

_____

_____

What is the hardest part of gathering information about your child's friends and activities?

_____

_____

_____

_____

What strategies have you found to be most successful for gathering information?

_____

_____

_____

_____

SANE Guidelines for Limit Setting

Identifying Consequences and Monitoring Questions

OVERVIEW AND RATIONALE

When behavioral theory was initially applied to helping troubled families, it was hoped that positive changes in families could be made exclusively by increasing contingent positive reinforcement for positive behavior. This approach was unsuccessful in part because of coercive behaviors among family members: when there is family conflict, family members use coercive behaviors to reduce aversive events. However, aversive family events are in the eye of the beholder and can include parents' requests for the child to follow rules, do chores, and the like. Children may react negatively until the parent relents and withdraws the expectation. It became clear that to help families out of the coercion trap, it was necessary to support their limit-setting skills so parents could sustain their leadership role.

There are considerable benefits to setting limits for children and adolescents. First and foremost is that, through following reasonable limits and rules in the family, children learn the critical skill of self-regulation. Self-regulation is the ability to do what is right for the group rather than prioritize one's own wishes. This critical skill is at the core of education (e.g., doing homework), success in personal relationships, and success at work. The second benefit to children is that skillful limit setting reduces negativity, tension, and conflict in families, which benefits all family members. Effective limits will reduce problem behaviors and strongly benefit the long-term adjustment and happiness of the child. Finally, clear and consistent limits and structure in the family provide children and adolescents with a sense of security and predictability within which to develop.

Skillful limit setting and positive behavior support fit together. One metaphor that is useful for many families is to see limits and rules as the boundaries of the road on which children and adolescents travel to adulthood and to see that positive behavior support provides the motivation to travel this road (see Figure 9).

Several benefits to parents come from increasing their limit-setting skills with their children or adolescents. Aside from the benefits to children described earlier, improving these skills will lead parents to feel respected by their children, will reduce stress in family life, and will ultimately improve the parent–child relationship, with adults functioning in an appropriate leadership role.

Two features of rules and limits are critical for success. First, the rules and limits must be clear to the child and reasonable for the child's developmental level. Second, the consequences should be SANE—that is, (S) Small is better, (A) Avoid punishing yourself, (N) Nonabusive action works better, and (E) Effective consequences work better. These points are discussed later in this session. SANE describes principles for parents to consider in terms of how they use consequences.

The myths that often guide the consequences that parents use have deleterious effects on the child or adolescent and weaken the family in the long run. One common myth is that the punishment should fit the crime. Thus the more a problem behavior upsets a parent, the more dramatic and severe the consequence. Although this approach may work for some families when the child has low levels of problem behavior, it is decidedly unsuccessful for daily living for most parents. For adolescents, a 3-month grounding is an example of a consequence that may work in a small number of families but will likely not work in most. One reason that such consequences are unsuccessful is that parents are unable to follow through. Another reason is that it is difficult to use other consequences once everything has been taken away from a child or adolescent. The SANE guidelines were designed to help parents understand the principles behind effective limits and consequences. By and large, small consequences are better than large ones for long-term behavior change.

To continue with the theme of monitoring, in this session we also provide a role-play activity that supports parents' skills at asking their children questions. The way in which parents ask their children about their behavior or experiences often turns *off* the faucet of information. Given that monitoring and limit setting go hand in hand, asking the right monitoring questions is an effective tool to help parents decide which limits to prioritize.

SUGGESTED TOOLS

➤ Handout on the SANE guidelines

➤ Handout on rules and consequences

➤ Whiteboard, chalkboard, or large sheets of paper

SESSION OBJECTIVES

➤ Suggest that parents focus on the limits and consequences they might want to use.

FIGURE 9   Parental limit setting and positive behavior support in the path of life.

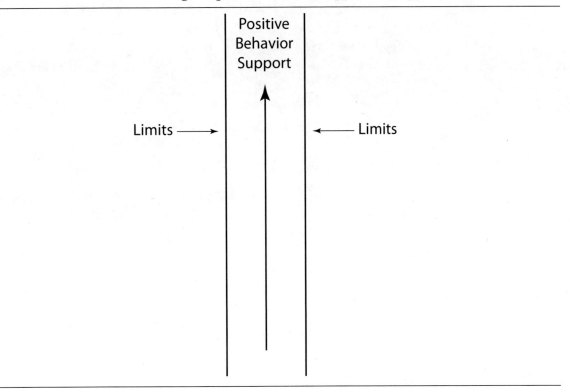

> ➤ Role-play monitoring questions.

> ➤ Discuss with parents how to practice at home generating rules and consequences.

COMMON PITFALLS AND SOLUTIONS

Motivation

We suggest moving slowly on limit setting to avoid eliciting resistance up front to effective limit-setting practices. We make this recommendation because in our experience limit setting tends to evoke the most emotion in parents and relates most strongly to how they were parented. There is, of course, no wrong way to set limits, except when it results in abuse to the child or adolescent or, less frequently, the parent. We have found that if the parents agree and understand the SANE guidelines, then it is far easier to discuss specific consequences, such as time-out, corrective consequences, and privilege removal.

Tailoring

The Session 5 exercise What Kind of Parent Are You? may be useful to review as you tailor limit setting for the parent. The exercise will provide some insight about the most effective way to tailor this information to the needs of the family. How this process is approached will vary if the parent self-identifies as a sibling parent or a parent-as-boss. Both styles have their advantages, disadvantages, and underlying emotional dynamics. For example, for a parent who wishes to remain a friend to his or her child, there may be tremendous anxiety and fear that setting a limit will distance the child at best or ruin the relationship at worst. The parent-as-boss may worry that if he or she is too lenient, the child or adolescent won't learn what he or she needs to know to be successful. Stepparents may feel underlying confusion and emotions regarding their role in limit setting. In general, we recommend that stepparents take a supportive role to the biological parent, at least initially when new limits and consequences are being set. In the interest of reducing the total number of sessions, it may be unnecessary to go through all the material in Sessions 5 and 6 for some families. Parents with a great deal of skill and judgment may not need the session on SANE guidelines, and they can jump directly to time-out, privilege removal, or whatever consequence is likely to be effective.

Structuring Sessions to Reduce Barriers

Session 6 is often conducted with Session 5, and it may be necessary to give parents feedback on limits or rules that are unreasonable (e.g., 4 hours of chores per day). It's important to do it in a way that keeps parents engaged in the limit-setting discussion and motivated to set more realistic rules and consequences. It is helpful to have parents read the SANE guidelines out loud, to keep the session active, and to reduce the amount of lecturing time. Then ask the parents to ask questions or make comments on how the guidelines would apply to their own family. This approach helps reduce parental resistance to feedback about their limit setting and places them in a self-evaluation role.

SETTING THE AGENDA

Good to see you again. Today we are going to dive into the core set of ideas that help parents decide what limits to focus on and that enable them to have a consequence ready if their child does not follow the rules. Before we begin, has anything happened in the past week that we should discuss before talking more about limit setting?

If anything has happened that would affect parents' skill development during the session, it should be briefly addressed, and they should be asked if they are ready to continue the work started in the previous session.

I have planned that we would cover the following today (write on a piece of paper, whiteboard, etc., so the parents can see the list):

- Review any past work with the parents.

- Discuss SANE guidelines.

- Discuss rules and limit setting.

- Discuss questions that help with monitoring.

- Discuss the home practice experiment.

Does this seem doable for today? Is there anything else you would like to address?

REVIEW OF SESSION 5

Last week we practiced monitoring as our family management skill and active listening (encouraging and paraphrasing) as our communication skill. Before we get started with any new topics, I would like to answer any questions you have about what we covered last week.

Ask parents to discuss active listening and review how they were able to practice the skills with their children during the week. Review any barriers to parents' active listening skills. Review the four Cs and discuss any barriers parents encountered during the week.

To help remember what we talked about last time, let's go through this short review.

Four Cs Review Activity

1. What are the four Cs of parental monitoring?

    - Clear rules

    - Consistency

    - Checking up

    - Communication

2. Which of the following statements is an effective way to begin a talk with your child about making a change in his or her behavior (the last two statements are the most effective):

    - "I've noticed that you never listen when I talk."

    - "You seem to be lazy when it comes to homework."

    - "I'd like to talk to you about getting chores done."

    - "We need to talk about your homework routine."

3. Good active listening skills require you to:

    - Show understanding

    - Practice patience

    - Emphasize positive behavior

    - Summarize what your child said

FAMILY MANAGEMENT SKILL: SETTING LIMITS WITH CHILDREN AND ADOLESCENTS

➤ Provide rationale for setting limits.

➤ Set up house rules.

➤ Discuss consistent limits.

➤ Identify guidelines for setting limits.

➤ Learn to gather information with effective questions.

Why Set Limits?

All children misbehave or push the rules every now and then. It takes time for them to learn the boundaries for acceptable behavior, particularly when the boundaries are not clear. Consistency is the key to setting effective limits. When children misbehave, it's up to parents, teachers, and other adults to set reasonable and consistent limits.

Having clear limits helps children understand the parents' expectations for their behavior. When children understand these expectations, they are more able to follow the rules and demonstrate positive behavior. Setting clear and consistent limits provides a structure to help your child behave positively and successfully.

Benefits for Parents

· *Increased cooperation and respect from children*

· *More positive behavior from children*

· *Increased likelihood of a well-functioning home*

· *Reduced stress for parents*

· *Improved parent–child relationship*

Benefits for Children

· *Children learn to cooperate with others and practice self-control.*

· *Not setting limits can lead to coercive family interactions that are unpleasant for all and harmful to children's development.*

· *When children can understand what you want, they're more likely to behave.*

· *When you set limits, it reduces the likelihood of long-term behavior problems.*

· *Children feel a sense of security when the limits are well understood and there is daily consistency in family routines.*

Setting limits and offering incentives are equally important for guiding your child's life. It's important for parents to set rules so that expectations of behavior are clear. Rules are great, especially when your kids follow them, but the big question is What do I do when my kids don't follow the rules? During the upcoming weeks, we'll provide information about consequences that work.

If you have difficulty setting limits with your child, you're not alone. It's a common problem for other parents, too. The relationship between children and parents changes over time, and as children mature, previously used consequences are no longer appropriate. Right now, I'd like you to assess yourself in terms of what kinds of challenges you face in disciplining your child.

Remember, all children need clear guidelines. The first step of limit setting is to establish **clear rules** *that your child understands.*

The second step is to develop—in advance—a good list of **consequences** *for your child's problem behaviors. In the third step,* **use the consequences consistently** *if your child crosses the limits, or in other words, when [she] breaks the rules you've set for [her]. Being consistent about consequences is as important as using incentives.*

LIMIT SETTING: QUESTIONS OF THE WEEK

Many parents struggle with setting limits for a variety of reasons. Some parents worry about how their children will respond to limits and therefore avoid setting consistent limits with them. Other parents set too many limits. Let's go over the questions on Handout 5E, which you filled out at home last week.

If parents didn't fill out the form at home, give them time to think about the questions before reviewing.

QUESTIONS TO ASK PARENTS

> ➤ What is the hardest part of setting limits with your child?

> ➤ What strategies have you used to address this problem?

> ➤ What is the hardest part of gathering information about your child's friends and activities?

> ➤ What strategies have you found to be most successful when gathering information?

HOUSE RULES

Ask parents what types of rules and consequences they use in their family. Make a list of all the rules and consequences.

Before you can use consequences (which we'll talk about next week), you need to establish what rules you want in your house and develop a plan to introduce and monitor those rules.

On Handout 6A, I'd like you to generate one rule that will help you supervise your child when [she] is away from home and two rules for home behavior. The rules you make should be for troublesome behaviors that you don't think will change using a behavior plan or that are serious concerns. Clear rules work well with serious behaviors because children often will comply when they know they face a consequence for noncooperation.

Make rules for the most important concern you have about your child. For example, if your child isn't coming home on time for dinner, your rule might be Be home each night by 5:30 p.m.

Home practice for parents this session includes tracking the rules they generate. Go over Handout 6A. At the end of the session is a reminder to track these rules.

CONSISTENCY

*Consistency is the second step in effective limit setting. If you want your rules to have an impact on your child's behavior, you need to be consistent. Being consistent means providing a consequence **each time** a rule is broken or not followed. All of us have problems being consistent. What gets in the way of being consistent?*

Have parents generate a list of things that interfere with being consistent and discuss the list. An example might be *coming up with a meaningful consequence.* Discuss possible solutions to the examples of things that interfere.

GUIDELINES FOR SETTING LIMITS

*Setting limits effectively requires more than being consistent. Parents can follow certain guidelines when setting limits with their children, both older adolescents and younger children. We call this the **SANE** approach to setting limits, which is outlined in Handout 6B.*

Ask parents to read the items in Handout 6C, then decide why the consequence does or does not fit the SANE guidelines for setting limits. This exercise will give them practice using the guidelines and give you information about their understanding of the guidelines.

FAMILY COMMUNICATION SKILL: QUESTIONS THAT HELP WITH MONITORING

Ask parents how they currently gather information about their child. Acknowledge that many times parents are already practicing the skills being presented.

You are your child's most valuable resource. Your ability to be a good resource depends on the information you have about your [daughter], both at home and in other settings. As children move through school, the number of friends, teachers, and activities in [her] life increases, and it becomes much harder to have direct knowledge about what's going on with [her]. It's important to have effective strategies for gathering information that don't totally rely on what your child tells you.

Adolescents are protecting their privacy and independence at a time when you need good information about their lives. Younger children lack the communication skills necessary to provide information about daily interactions at school.

*There are three common ways parents get information about their children. One is **tracking**. Another is getting information by **networking** with adults, such as teachers, parents, and coaches who are involved with their children in other settings. One other common way parents get information about their children is through **questioning**. We've covered tracking and networking, so today we'll focus on questioning.*

Questioning

As you have probably learned, the way you ask your child about [her] life affects the quality of information you receive. Questions that hint of blame or disapproval tend to lead children away from sharing useful information. Questions that show interest and concern encourage your child to talk and give you good information that tells you what your child is doing when you're not around and how [she] thinks and feels about the world. Let's look at some typical questions parents ask their kids and decide which questions will lead to useful information.

Ask the parents to read the questions on Handout 6D and decide which are examples of questions that will get useful information from their child without causing a fight or argument.

Wrong Way/Right Way to Ask Questions

Read through the section called Things to Remember When Questioning, which is at the bottom of Handout 6D.

As a brief exercise, if both parents are present, ask them to be "parent" and "child" and take turns practicing the parent role. If only one parent is in the session, take the role of "parent" first to demonstrate and build parent confidence. First, have the "parent" practice asking informal questions of the "child" about his or her day at school. Then practice the wrong way, with the "child" reacting to the wrong way. Next have them do it the right way. Each parent should have an opportunity to take each role. Remind parents that this is a good opportunity to use the active listening skills taught earlier.

HOME PRACTICE

I'd like you to practice questioning. There are three parts to this home practice. First, think of two questions to ask your child, then listen in a way that will give you as much information as possible. Review the Handout 6D suggestions before asking the questions and completing Handout 6E.

Second, as we talked about earlier, I'd like you to track the house rules you came up with. A form for tracking your child's response to the house rules can be found on Handout 6F. Third, I'd like you to take some time and answer the questions on Handout 6G about getting information from your child.

Behavior Rule 1: _____

How to check: _____

Behavior Rule 2: _____

How to check: _____

Behavior Rule 3: _____

How to check: _____

S = Small Is Better

It is better to give a small consequence consistently than a large consequence inconsistently. Small consequences are easier to provide. For example, a 1-day restriction is better than 2 weeks. A short time-out is better than a long, unsuccessful time-out. A long, severe restriction may put the child in a no-win situation that actually leads to more problem behavior.

A = Avoid Punishing Yourself

Some consequences we pick for our children punish parents as well. A 2-week restriction may be punishing for a parent to enforce. Often, special events during the long restriction cause desperate pleas for leniency, arguments, and so forth. Having an angry child around the house for 2 weeks can be agony for parents.

N = Nonabusive Action Works Better

Abusive actions create bad feelings and give children the wrong message about how to communicate with others. The best way to avoid abusive actions is to avoid giving consequences when you are upset.

E = Effective Consequences Work Better

Consequences that are under your control and that are not rewarding are effective. The most effective consequences simply remove positive activities.

From *Everyday Parenting: A Professional's Guide to Building Family Management Skills,* © 2012 by T. J. Dishion, E. A. Stormshak, and K. A. Kavanagh, Champaign, IL: Research Press (www.researchpress.com, 800-519-2707).

*Read the consequences below and discuss them as they relate to the SANE guidelines. Put a **Y** (for yes) by those that follow the SANE guidelines and an **N** (for no) by those that don't. For each item that you mark **N**, explain which guideline(s) the consequence violates.*

_____   1. Parent drives the child to and from school for a month as a consequence for being suspended from school.

_____   2. Parent slaps the child across the face because the child swore at her.

_____   3. Parent restricts the child from any contact with friends.

_____   4. Parent takes the child's skateboard away for 2 days because the child is not doing homework.

_____   5. Parent restricts phone use for 1 day as a consequence for coming home late from a friend's house.

_____   6. Parent criticizes the child for stupidity and laziness when he brings home a report card with Cs and Ds.

_____   7. Parent gives a 30-minute work chore of cleaning the top of the stove for a child's lying about where he or she has been.

_____   8. Parent puts 2-year-old child on a time-out for 10 minutes after she knocked down her brother's block tower.

From *Everyday Parenting: A Professional's Guide to Building Family Management Skills,* © 2012 by T. J. Dishion, E. A. Stormshak, and K. A. Kavanagh, Champaign, IL: Research Press (www.researchpress.com, 800-519-2707).

*Which questions do you think will get useful information about your child? Place an **I** on the line preceding those questions. Which do you think will result in angry feelings for both you and your child? Place an **A** on the line preceding those questions.*

_____A_____ 1. "What? I suppose you don't have any homework again?" (disapproving tone of voice)

_____I_____ 2. "What kinds of homework assignments are you getting these days?"

_____ 3. "You're not seeing John again, are you?"

_____ 4. "What were you thinking, talking to the teacher like that?" (irritated tone of voice)

_____ 5. "I'm afraid to ask whom you went to the mall with today."

_____ 6. "Whom did you see at the mall today?"

_____ 7. "I haven't talked to you for a while. Whom are you spending time with these days?"

_____ 8. "Were you really upset when you were talking to the teacher?"

_____ 9. "Whom did you play with today at school?"

_____ 10. "What did you do when you were over at Sarah's house?"

Things to Remember When Questioning

Wrong Way

- Use a negative tone

- Accuse

- Interrupt

- Use sarcasm

Right Way

- Choose a good time

- Use a neutral or positive tone

- Show interest or understanding

- Paraphrase

From *Everyday Parenting: A Professional's Guide to Building Family Management Skills,* © 2012 by T. J. Dishion, E. A. Stormshak, and K. A. Kavanagh, Champaign, IL: Research Press (www.researchpress.com, 800-519-2707).

Questions I asked my child:

1. _____

2. _____

Did I ...	Question 1	Question 2
Choose a good time to ask?	☐ Yes ☐ No	☐ Yes ☐ No
Use a neutral or positive tone?	☐ Yes ☐ No	☐ Yes ☐ No
Show interest or understanding?	☐ Yes ☐ No	☐ Yes ☐ No
Paraphrase?	☐ Yes ☐ No	☐ Yes ☐ No

What I learned:

1. _____

2. _____

Use this chart to track whether your child is currently following your house rules. Use a plus sign (+) to show that the house rule was followed. Use a minus sign (−) to show that the rule was broken.

Week of: _____

Rule	Sun.	Mon.	Tues.	Wed.	Thurs.	Fri.	Sat.

Clear Rule 1: _____

Consequences: _____

Clear Rule 2: _____

Consequences: _____

Clear Rule 3: _____

Consequences: _____

What is the hardest part about getting useful information from your child? (This can be something you do or something your child does, or it can be a situation, such as no time or no privacy.)

_____

_____

_____

_____

What have you done to address this problem?

_____

_____

_____

_____

Proactive Limit-Setting Plan

Giving Consequences and Ignoring Mild Problem Behavior

OVERVIEW AND RATIONALE

This session focuses on two interrelated facets of limit setting: giving consequences and ignoring trivial problem behaviors. These two family management skills are inextricably related. For parents to effectively give consequences, they need to choose their battles wisely. When they have chosen their focus, in order to be consistent and to follow through, they need to ignore the trivia and stick with the game plan. Although we know there is no winning or losing in family relationships, it is possible to think about parents "winning" a limit-setting exchange in that parents have the last word and the child respects their leadership. If the child "wins," in the long run, he or she loses. When children succeed in coercively avoiding limits, these behaviors spill over into other areas of their lives and can be the source of failure in relationships, in academic learning, and in developing satisfying work and recreational activities. For parents to effectively assume and maintain leadership, it must be understood that they have the child's best interests at heart and are compassionate, fair, and reasonable in the limits they set and the consequences they impose for problem behavior.

Time-out is the cornerstone of SANE guidelines for limit setting and consequences. It is not widely known that time-out was developed with young adolescents who had problems with aggression. Thus time-out can be a useful parent tool from early childhood (as early as age 2) through early adolescence. However, the framing of time-out will vary considerably with the developmental level of the child and the ecology of the family. Time-out is most appropriate for interpersonal forms of misbehavior that involve conflict, escalation, or disrespect in daily family living. Successful time-outs depend on (1) the parents' ability to make a clear and proactive limit-setting plan, (2) the parents' self-regulation when responding to problem behavior, and (3) the parents' ability to ignore aspects of the child's behavior that potentially disrupt her or his ability to carry out the plan. For example, if the child says, "I don't care, I like to go to time-out!" when given a time-out consequence, it is best for everyone to ignore this provocation. When a child comes out of time-out and says or does things that are mildly provocative, it is best not to respond to the provocation but to wipe the slate clean, ignore the trivia, and focus on the fact that the child cooperated with the time-out. It's useful for parents to know that when a child goes to time-out, the child learns about the need to consider the wishes of others in the family. Small consequences are better than large consequences because parents are more likely to consistently use them. This strategy makes it possible for the entire five-step learning sequence to occur, which is essential for effective limit setting.

> Parent requests behavior change → child is uncooperative → parent labels and gives consequence → child accepts → parent is neutral or positive.

Using this sequence as the dominant limit-setting interaction will benefit the child and the parent in the ways discussed in Session 6.

Time-out is not for every family. There are some reasons why time-out may not be successful in a family. First and foremost is environment. In a crowded living situation, there may be no place the child can go to remove himself or herself from social contact and reinforcement. Second, the parents may not agree about time-out but potentially do agree about another possible consequence, such as a privilege removal or corrective consequence. This session covers all these types of consequences, and the therapist should tailor the limit-setting strategy to fit the family's needs. Privilege removal has the advantage of being nonconfrontational in that the parent selects a privilege that is within her or his control and removes it, contingently, when the child or adolescent is uncooperative. That is the end of the story, and the family moves on to the next moment in their daily life. One example of this kind of consequence is the action of a petite mother of a 6-foot-tall adolescent male who was intimidating in limit-setting episodes. Mom selected skateboard removal for 1 hour when he was disrespectful. This was a successful strategy for this family overall, and it helped the 15-year-old adolescent learn respect for his mother.

The key to success in limit setting is having a proactive plan. For this reason, we develop a plan and a backup plan in case the original one does not work. For example, if a child does not go to time-out, then the parent removes a privilege and moves on with the day, remains neutral and constructive, and does not criticize or hold a grudge for the rest of the day. This is a difficult task for most parents because the tendency is to respond emotionally to the negative interaction. Parents should practice having backup plans and following through with those plans. Role-play and rehearsal in the session will greatly improve the family's success in limit setting. Rehearsing the plan will provide a guided success experience that can increase the parents' sense of self-efficacy and make limit setting seem feasible even though some anxiety may ensue.

One major aspect of a successful plan is for the therapist to be knowledgeable about the history of the parents and child relevant to limit setting and to understand previous barriers and parents' strengths in leadership.

SUGGESTED TOOLS

➤ Handout on the SANE guidelines (as a reminder)

➤ Videotape on time-out or limit setting

➤ Worksheet on rules and consequences

➤ Whiteboard, chalkboard, or large sheets of paper

SESSION OBJECTIVES

➤ Establish a limit-setting plan for at least one behavior.

➤ Collaboratively develop a backup plan for the family.

➤ Role-play and rehearse the limit-setting plan, including backup plan.

➤ Role-play ignoring trivial problem behavior.

➤ Prepare parent for successful home practice experiment.

COMMON PITFALLS AND SOLUTIONS

Motivation

One of the problems with working with a time-out plan is dealing with past failures. When time-out was first introduced in the 1960s and 1970s, parents rarely had exposure to the strategy, and therefore it seemed novel and interesting. Currently, the use of time-out is widespread, and more often than not, parents will have tried time-out without success. In these cases, unsuccessful time-out experiences should be broken down and discussed in terms of which aspects worked and which didn't. If past successes can be identified, they build parents' readiness to try again. It's also important to acknowledge that time-out is a challenge to implement well and requires rehearsal and coaching to be successful, especially with one's own child. In addition, there are two significant motivational styles. Some parents want only to punish misbehavior, and they quickly escalate and become emotional if the child does not cooperate, feeding into the coercion trap. This situation is best dealt with up front by having the parent identify the danger and make a proactive plan to avoid this reaction. Information from the What Kind of Parent Are You? exercise in Session 5 that identified discipline styles can also be used to objectify this style and enable the parent to collaboratively work on strategies. Second, some parents are anxious about and avoidant of conflict with the child, and they will be challenged to execute a limit-setting plan when it comes time to give a consequence. Again, up-front identification of this understandable tendency is important. It is also important to start slow and encourage the parent to follow through with the plan, even though it may be initially uncomfortable. To build on the parents' strengths, it may be helpful to find out about situations in which the parents have successfully overcome fear and anxiety in other aspects of their life.

Tailoring

In tailoring this session, it is more productive to have the parent be successful in a small limit-setting encounter than to deal with a more challenging problem behavior. Thus the therapist needs to help the parents assess their own strengths and to set up a proactive limit-setting plan that is realistic for those parents in the current living situation. It is also essential to tailor the proactive limit-setting plan to the parenting situation. For example, if parents in a blended family are having trouble agreeing on limit setting, the plan may be for the biological parent to be the one who executes the limit-setting plan for his or her child while the stepparent supports the biological parent in his or her effort, whether successful or not.

Structuring Sessions to Reduce Barriers

Given that this session is action packed in terms of ensuring that the parent is well prepared to try a limit-setting plan for the coming week, it is especially advisable that the therapist structure the session up front. The therapist can forewarn the parent that it is important to accomplish certain goals so that if other issues come up, they will be put on the back burner to discuss after the role-plays.

SETTING THE AGENDA

Greetings. We have a lot to do today because we are going to work together to come up with a limit-setting plan that will work for your family that you can experiment with next week. I want you to be successful, so I'm going to work with you to rehearse and problem-solve.

I have planned that we would cover the following today (write on a piece of paper, whiteboard, etc., so the parents can see the list):

- Review the limit-setting plan you worked on last week.

- Suggest a consequence that will fit your family.

- Practice the limit-setting plan and backup plan.

- Practice ignoring the trivial problem behaviors.

- Discuss the home practice experiment.

Does this seem doable for today? Is there anything else you would like to address? To make sure we get through this and that you feel prepared, I may ask that we put other issues that come up on the back burner to be talked about at the end of our meeting today or the next time we meet.

REVIEW OF SESSION 6

> *During this meeting, we'll continue our discussion about setting limits with children. But first, let's review the work you did at home during the past week.*

If you worked with the family on positive behavior support, review the incentive plan as you do each week. Problem-solve obstacles and make revisions to the plan as necessary.

> *Part of your home practice was to use questioning, the communication skill we talked about last week.*

Ask parents if they brought in their practice sheets and review the information using the content of the following questions as a guide. If they did not bring their sheet, then the following questions are useful for discussing their home practice.

QUESTIONS TO ASK PARENTS

➤ What kinds of questions did you ask your child?

➤ Did you get any surprising information?

➤ Were you able to listen without interrupting?

➤ Did you choose a good time to ask the questions?

➤ Did you remember to use a neutral or positive tone?

➤ Did you show interest or understanding?

➤ Did you paraphrase the response you heard from your child?

➤ The last two parts of home practice for the previous session were to track your house rules and to answer the questions of the week on Handout 6G. What did you find out from the tracking? If you didn't track, what interfered with tracking? If you didn't get a chance to ask your child questions, try to do so in the coming week.

It is important to process what the parents found out while tracking house rules. Some parents will learn that a rule they set was never followed or that one of the three rules they made was unclear. They may also learn that their child's behavior improves when rules are explicit and compliance is tracked.

FAMILY MANAGEMENT SKILL: GIVING CONSEQUENCES

Objectives

➤ Create a plan for giving consequences.

➤ Identify types of consequences.

➤ Communicate limits to your child.

➤ Learn when to ignore.

Plan for Setting Consequences

*The best way to stay consistent as a parent is to have a **consequences plan** when rules are broken. When you develop a plan, to be successful, it should reflect your strengths and weaknesses as a parent. For example, if you're having a problem with consistency, choose a consequence that is totally under your control.*

***Consequences** can be broken down into four types:*

- *Corrective actions*
- *Loss of privileges*
- *Work chores*
- *Time-out*

The type of consequence you use will depend on the behavior and age of your child. Explanations of the four types of consequences are on Handout 7A.

Using the SANE Guidelines to Develop a Plan

Now let's use Handout 7B and apply the SANE guidelines to develop a plan for the three rules you made and tracked last week. Or, if you decided other rules were more important during the week, write those down and make consequences for those rules.

Giving a Consequence

Now that you have your plan, let's talk about putting it into action. Giving a consequence in the heat of the moment can be challenging. Often, when we're angry, the things we say and do are automatic and not always the best choice. This is where it helps to catch a problem early, before you've had to give several warnings.

Handout 7C includes four things to do when giving a consequence to avoid bigger problems. Follow the steps in a calm but firm tone of voice.

USING TIME-OUT WITH YOUNGER CHILDREN

Time-out is the consequence of choice for young children. The basic approach is to interrupt children's misbehavior by removing them from the social situation and placing them in a boring place where they can't disrupt others or get attention.

The Benefits of Time-Out

➤ Effective—because it immediately stops disruptive behavior

➤ Easy to use

➤ Nonabusive to the child

➤ Does not punish the parent

➤ Safe because it provides a cooling-off period for parent and child

➤ Gives children an opportunity to change their behavior without prolonged punishment

➤ Gives children a fresh chance at behaving well

➤ Can be modified to fit a family's needs

➤ Teaches children self-control

➤ When used consistently, teaches child that parent "means business"

➤ Sets up a pattern of discipline that both child and parent understand and know how to use

➤ Reduces the tendency to use yelling and/or physical punishment

➤ Results in fewer power struggles

Time-Out Guidelines Through Privilege Removal

➤ Time-out is short, starting at 1 minute.

➤ Add 1 minute at a time, adding up to 5 minutes (for a total of 6 minutes).

➤ If child does not go to time-out after adding maximum minutes, remove a privilege for 30 minutes to 1 hour.

Making Time-Out Work

Various forms of time-out have been tested over the years. Some forms work really well; others don't.

➤ Our form is short (starts at 1 minute, depending on the age of the child).

➤ A brief, 1-minute time-out may be all that is needed.

➤ For young children, add up to 5 more minutes in time-out (with 6 as the maximum) if the child refuses to go.

➤ If at 6 minutes the child still refuses, we simply remove a privilege for 30 minutes. This teaches the child that it's better to go to time-out for a few minutes than to lose 30 minutes of a privilege they value.

➤ Time-out involves no physical contact and no yelling, arguing, or other emotional behavior, at least not for the adults. After a while the child will be calm, too.

When you start, use time-out for a simple behavior, such as not follow-ing directions. Not minding (noncompliance, not cooperating) is a good first behavior for time-out because this behavior tends to be a problem for most kids every single day. Make sure you give good clear directions. Make it easy on yourself and your child by giving [her] directions for simple behaviors, such as hanging up [her] coat, putting shoes away, closing the door—things that take only a minute to do and can be done right away. Save complicated behaviors (going to bed, doing homework) for later. Then combine complex behaviors with encouragement (maybe include them on the incentive chart). Refer to Handout 7D for a detailed sequence of behaviors related to administering time-out.

PREDICTING PROBLEMS

Most children will test the new limits, and it's important to remember that when you start using time-out or anytime you make a change to discipline routines. The time-out response often results in an increase in problems for a short time.

When you first use time-out, you may see an increase in noncompliance while your child finds out if you really will follow through. Saying that time-out doesn't bother them is another common strategy children use. In fact, they may say "Time-out is fun" or "I like time-out." The novelty will soon wear off, so stay focused. Don't get pulled into a power struggle. Just follow through with the consequence and then cool off. Don't measure the effectiveness of time-out by the kind of reaction your child has to it.

FAMILY COMMUNICATION SKILL: STAYING NEUTRAL AND IGNORING MISBEHAVIOR

The success of your plan for setting limits depends on how well you communicate limits to your children. **Giving neutral forewarning** *can prevent a lot of problems. Staying neutral when you give the consequence will help avoid an argument.*

When you go home, discuss the rules and consequences you made with your child. We suggest you use this formula for talking to your child. Remember to wait for a good time to bring up rules and consequences. Don't try to do it if your child has misbehaved or if you are stressed, angry, or upset.

Rules and Consequences Formula

1. "I want to review a couple of important rules with you."

2. "Whenever you break one of these rules, you'll get one of these consequences."

3. "Do you have any questions about how this will work?"

It's equally important to preview time-out for younger children. It's a good idea to explain and demonstrate what will happen when the child is asked to do something and doesn't do it. Most young children have no problem pretending to say no and then going through the process. If a child doesn't want to role-play, parents should still make sure the child understands what time-out is before implementing it the first time.

IGNORING MISBEHAVIOR

Ignoring misbehavior involves not responding in any way to something annoying or distressing that someone else says or does. Often, when we react to the negative things our kids do, it just reinforces their behavior. Ignoring their behavior makes it less likely that it will happen again in the future.

Arguing with your child does not end the discussion; it prolongs it. Ignoring complaints, whines, and expressions of anger makes it less likely that you will get sucked into arguments. Ignoring is useful when your child is doing something that is annoying, attention getting, or argumentative. Hurtful, dangerous, or aggressive behaviors, however, should not be ignored. Ignoring is a key parenting skill for younger children and can be used when children are whining, crying, pouting, or making faces at their parents. It is common to forget that ignoring can still be useful with adolescents for many of the same behaviors (whining, pouting, moodiness).

*Ignoring is an **active**, not a passive, process. While ignoring, you should be on the lookout for the moment when your child stops the annoying behavior and begins to show more appropriate behavior. At that point, you should give your child positive verbal support for positive behavior.*

Ask parents to discuss the pros and cons they see in ignoring little things their children do. Then have them brainstorm the things their children do that they might ignore. Refer to examples given on Handout 7E.

HOME PRACTICE

If parents have been working on an incentive plan:

This time, I'd like you to continue to work on your incentive plan and practice praising completion of targeted behaviors, along with giving incentives.

This week you can present the consequences of not following the rules to your child. Use the tracking form on Handout 6F to keep track of how often your rules are followed and how often you have to give a consequence. If your child doesn't break any of the rules, remember to give positive verbal support.

For younger children:

This week you can present time-out to your child and practice it when [she] doesn't comply with your requests. Remember to also praise compliance each time it happens.

Ask parents to review Handout 7F before starting to use time-out. Keep incentives separate from setting limits.

If your teen has earned [her] incentives, [she] gets them, regardless of the rules [she] broke. Keep up the hard work.

I'd also like you to answer the questions on Handout 7G about changing your child's behavior.

Corrective Actions

A corrective action should be used when your child needs to repair the damage caused by previous misbehavior. For example, your child has some friends over after school, and they mess up the kitchen. The appropriate consequence would be to clean the kitchen and restore it to its original condition. Your preschooler left toys all over the floor. The appropriate consequence is for the child to put the toys away.

Loss of Privileges

Your child should have some privileges he **or she** enjoys that can be removed if necessary. For example, if you get a report from school that your son has not done homework, TV privileges can be withheld each night until homework is completed. (Taking away TV privileges will not be effective for a child who does not normally watch a lot of television.) Many children own electronic devices, such as iPods and handheld computer games. These can be removed for a short time as a loss of privilege or consequence for misbehavior.

Work Chores

Chores are appropriate for older children and can be used as a consequence. It isn't necessary to make work chores unbearable, but they should not be rewarding. The best work chores do not require complicated skills and are easy to check (for example, pulling weeds, cleaning bathroom tiles, washing windows, sweeping the patio). Brief work chores are the most effective. For example, a 1-hour work chore when your child lies about where she has been is effective and SANE.

Time-Out

Use a time-out when the best solution is to remove your child from a situation. For example, if your daughter is teasing a younger sibling, send her to her room for a short period of time. Brief time-outs are much more effective and easier to reinforce than long ones. The time-out place should be boring but safe and have no rewards (in other words, no TV, radio, telephone, video games, or other people). Time-outs can be used more frequently with younger children.

Rule 1 (Home Behavior): _____

How to check: _____

Consequence: _____

Rule 2 (Home Behavior): _____

How to check: _____

Consequence: _____

Rule 3 (Out-of-Home Behavior): _____

How to check: _____

Consequence: _____

From *Everyday Parenting: A Professional's Guide to Building Family Management Skills,* © 2012 by T. J. Dishion, E. A. Stormshak, and K. A. Kavanagh, Champaign, IL: Research Press (www.researchpress.com, 800-519-2707).

In a calm but firm tone of voice …

1. Label the problem behavior in terms of your rule.

2. State the consequence clearly.

3. Avoid arguing.

4. Ignore trivia.

1. **Make a clear, direct request.**

   "The house rule is use an inside voice. Use your inside voice now, please."

   "I'm going to mow the lawn. Please put your toys in the box now."

2. **Provide no more than 10 seconds to allow cooperation.**

3. **If child doesn't cooperate, label the behavior and tell your child to go to time-out.**

   "That's not minding. Time-out for 1 minute."

   "You didn't put your toys away. Take a time-out now."

4. **Make sure the time-out place is safe and free from distractions and social attention.**

5. **If child does not go to time-out, add up to 5 minutes, giving child time to cooperate.**

   "That's 2 minutes."

   "That's 3 minutes."

   Continue until you reach 6 minutes.

6. **Set the timer for 1 to 6 minutes (depending on when you start time-out).**

   Set time-out according to the age of the child. Start at 1 minute for a 3-year-old and 3 minutes for a 5-year-old. Never begin time-out with more than 3 minutes for any age.

   For some children, a brief 1-minute time-out is all that is needed.

7. **Remove yourself from the scene.**

8. **Do not engage with your child while he or she is in time-out.**

9. **Stay neutral when time-out is over.**

   "Time's up!"

10. **Provide a cool-off period.**

    Take the temperature of the situation before deciding to repeat the direction.

    Is your child likely to comply? Are you able to calmly state the direction?

11. **Carry on.**

    Don't lecture or ask your child to apologize or promise never to do it again.

    When it's over, it's over—life goes on as it normally would.

If the Child Refuses to Go to Time-Out

1. **If the child does not go to time-out after adding maximum minutes, give a choice of time-out or privilege removal.**

   "Go to time-out now for 6 minutes or no (toy, activity) for 30 minutes."

2. **If child does not go to time-out, remove privilege.**

   "No [toy, activity] for 30 minutes."

3. **Remove yourself.**

Positive Examples

- Your son complains or makes a face when you ask him to do something, but he does what he is asked to do. You don't say anything about his complaint.

- Your son starts to argue with you. You turn away and start doing something else.

- Your daughter and son quarrel. You don't say anything.

- Your toddler screams every time he uses the toilet. You ignore the screaming and praise using the toilet properly.

Negative Examples

- Your son tells you that he hates his sister. You tell him that's no way to talk about his sister.

- You ask your daughter to do something for you, and, as she starts to do it, she makes a face. You tell her she needs to learn to be more respectful.

- Your daughter starts to argue with you, and you say, "I'm not going to argue with you."

- Your son does something annoying and you don't say anything to him, but you get angry and he can tell you are angry.

Keep up your encouragement system! Stay focused on the positive.

Step 1: Determine what misbehaviors (and when) result in time-out.

Step 2: Determine a list of possible privileges to remove.

Step 3: Determine and prepare time-out place.

Step 4: Explain time-out.

Step 5: Practice taking a time-out.

Step 6: Start using time-out.

Step 7: Make adjustments as necessary.

What's the hardest part about trying to get your child to change certain habits or behaviors?

_____

_____

_____

_____

What strategies have you found are successful for getting your child to make changes in his or her habits or behaviors?

_____

_____

_____

_____

Limit-Setting Challenges and Emotion Regulation

RATIONALE AND OVERVIEW

Serious problem behaviors in children and adolescents require considerable skill and emotional regulation in family management. The parenting demands associated with children who have multiple problem behaviors and emotional distress would overwhelm parents of well-adjusted children. Setting a fire, stealing family jewelry, lying about their behavior, and purposefully destroying property of a brother or sister are all examples of behavior that would provoke strong emotions in most parents. When children learn these behaviors, they become much more challenging to monitor and to effectively set limits for. The parents' reactions can spill over to disrupt the entire family, to break up marriages, and to lead to depression, defeat, and eventually caregivers giving up—or to conflict that goes out of control, resulting in abuse or the child leaving the family home. Successfully managing a problem behavior dramatically improves the outcome for the youth and the family.

In family situations such as these, it is prudent not to underestimate the challenges a parent faces. The paradox is this: the parent needs to do the opposite of what he or she feels in the situation—that is, the parent needs to react calmly with a plan when the tendency is to scream, yell, and seriously punish. As presented in the SANE guidelines, it is a myth that severe problem behavior demands severe consequences. In fact, severe punishment often elicits more problem behavior and conflict, as the coercion model would suggest.

Emotional reactions often stem from a blend of feelings: fear of what the behavior means and helplessness at not being able to alter the course of a child's adjustment or anger that a child has violated family rules and beliefs. It is because parents care about their families and their home that they react so intensely.

One way to prepare parents to manage these serious family events is to develop a proactive plan. Just knowing how one plans to respond removes some of the energy behind emotional reactions. There are two levels to a proactive

121

plan. One is to help parents troubleshoot and refine their limit-setting strategy to fit their child and family situation. The second is to make a plan by which they can manage their own reactions, which takes the pressure to react immediately off them. It is far better to respond well with a delay than to react immediately and decisively in a way that exacerbates the situation. This session is really about harm reduction and moving forward when children's emotions and behavior become challenging.

SUGGESTED TOOLS

➤ Handout on the SANE guidelines (as a reminder)

➤ Videotape on parents' emotional reactions to problem behavior (such as "Parenting in the Teenage Years," which is available from InterVision, 800-678-3455)

➤ Worksheet on rules and consequences and handouts

➤ Whiteboard, chalkboard, or large sheets of paper

SESSION OBJECTIVES

➤ Cover the CALM guidelines and role-play.

➤ Troubleshoot limit-setting problems.

➤ Create a limit-setting plan for other possible problem behaviors.

➤ Role-play possible scenario for the family.

COMMON PITFALLS AND SOLUTIONS

Motivation

One of the motivational issues for parents is that more serious problem behaviors, such as stealing, drug use, and lying, are covert in nature. Deception and avoidance of parent detection is the rule rather than the exception. It is often true that parents are not sure whether something is stolen or drugs are being used. In the early stages of these problem behaviors, parents may want to avoid a lapse in trust by accusing an innocent child of such behavior. It may be judicious for the parent to increase levels of monitoring in addition to having a plan if and when it becomes clear that the youth has stolen something, is using drugs, and the like. When a parent discovers that a child is engaging in a more serious problem behavior, it suggests that the usual parent–child trust has been violated. As such, the parent may introduce small consequences for "suspected lying" or "suspected unsupervised time in drug-using situations." Another common scenario is that a youth's problem behavior has special significance or makes a statement that is emotionally provocative. For example, stealing a new stepfather's special golf clubs and selling them will understandably provoke anger. Such behavior is unfortunately not as unusual as it may seem to the parents. This motivational context will benefit from validating the emotions involved and slowing down the reactions and, perhaps, from reframing the child's motivations for such behavior. Harm reduction involves getting perspective about the bigger picture of the family and the parents' long-term goals for themselves and their child.

Tailoring

It is particularly important to come prepared for this session with examples of likely scenarios that a parent may face with a child. In some ways this is predicting problems before they occur. For youths who are involved in deviant peer groups, smoking and other drug use are probably already occurring or are to be expected down the road. Parents need to be apprised of these risks based on research, not as a personal negative statement about their child. For example, it is similar to suggesting to a 40-year-old, overweight male who smokes and drinks that heart problems may be down the road and informing him of the symptoms.

Structuring Sessions to Reduce Barriers

If at least one of the parents is angry or resentful of a youth's behavior or tends to overreact in limit-setting situations, then this should be addressed during this session. A videotaped example or role-play may be used to assist parents with this process. Letting the parents see another parent reacting emotionally and the damage it does is a better way to enter into this topic than using a parent's current behavior as an example. The problem of parent overreaction is thus both objectified and normalized by watching one brief scenario.

SETTING THE AGENDA

Greetings. I'm very interested to hear how it went this past week with the new limit-setting plan for [Chris]. I want to go over that, and I also want us to talk about and prepare for other kinds of behaviors you may see in the future.

I have planned that we would cover the following today (write on a piece of paper, whiteboard, etc., so the parents can see the list):

• Review limit-setting plan you worked on last week.

• Troubleshoot problems with giving consequences.

• Learn about staying CALM when there is more serious problem behavior.

• Make a plan for consequences if more serious problem behavior occurs.

• Prepare for home practice experiment.

Is there anything else you would like to address today? To make sure we get through this and that you feel prepared, I may ask that we put other issues that come up on the back burner to be talked about at the end of our meeting today or the next time we meet.

REVIEW OF SESSION 7

Go over limit setting and behavior plans. Problem-solve any obstacles and provide ideas for improving existing plans.

Ideally you will have a copy of the parents' limit-setting plan to facilitate a good discussion. This tells them that their information is important to you and that you have taken the time to record and remember it. If they have brought their plan, use it for review.

Remember, last session we talked about the need for setting consequences for your child's behavior. Let's talk about the rules you set up with your child. I'd like you to answer some questions about how it went:

* *What rules did you set up?*

* *Did you present the rules to your child in a neutral tone?*

* *Were you able to check up on your child to see if the rules were followed? If not, what interfered?*

* *Did you set consequences when rules were broken?*

* *What obstacles prevented you from using a behavior plan or from setting limits?*

FAMILY MANAGEMENT SKILL: LIMIT-SETTING CHALLENGES

One difficulty in setting limits can be the impact of strong feelings about the type of consequences we give and the consistency with which we set limits.

*During this session, we'll discuss our family management skill, the **challenges of setting limits** for serious problem behaviors. Strong feelings often get in the way of how we deal with serious problem behaviors, such as aggression, lying, stealing, drug use, and sexual behavior. For our communication skill, we will learn how to use the **CALM** guidelines to deal with the strong emotions that often come with setting limits.*

SERIOUS PROBLEM BEHAVIORS

There are times when a child's behavior is serious enough to endanger [her] own life and/or the lives of others. For instance, these days it's risky for adolescents to be sexually active. Problem behavior, such as aggression or violence with siblings or peers, also can have a serious long-term effect on a child's adjustment. Youths who start using substances in adolescence are more at risk for developing serious drug or alcohol problems by adulthood. Stealing can lead to arrests and placement in detention. Truancy can re-

sult in school failure. Aggression with peers can lead to peer rejection at school and later affiliation with deviant peers in high school.

Circumstances for each family are different. You already may have found it necessary to set limits on more serious problem behavior. To be effective while dealing with these behaviors, parents need to set up rules that catch serious problems early. It's a mistake to wait for proof because by then it may be too late. The second mistake is to ignore risky situations in which more serious problem behavior can be learned and hidden. Handout 8A lists some warning signs to help parents catch problems early.

When rules are broken, a consequence should follow. Catching problems early makes it easier for parents to follow the SANE limit-setting guidelines.

It is a myth that these behaviors require severe punishment. The SANE guidelines apply to serious problem behaviors, too. Work chores, loss of privileges, and consequences that require correction of a behavior pattern can be effective with these more serious problems if they are applied consistently. It helps to have a plan.

LISTING CONSEQUENCES

Using Handout 8B, generate a list of consequences for problem behavior. List as many consequences as possible for each problem behavior and have them fit the SANE guidelines.

At the end of this exercise, make a statement about the kinds of consequences that should be avoided, particularly with respect to the short- and long-term effects on the child and the parent–child relationship:

This is a great list of consequences. We should end this discussion by acknowledging that some consequences that parents give are potentially harmful. For example, parents want to consider carefully how to react when their child tells them about [her] problem behavior. If you provide a severe consequence or react emotionally, you may stop communication. The first step when children tell you about problem behavior is to acknowledge their effort to be honest.

A negative feature of severe consequences is that some children will become secretive about their behavior, particularly adolescents. Children will go to great efforts to avoid being punished or admit problem behavior. When this happens, lying increases, and it becomes difficult to get accurate information and provide the needed supervision. To maintain a healthy relationship with your child, it is best to follow the SANE guidelines.

FAMILY COMMUNICATION SKILL: STAYING CALM WHEN SETTING LIMITS

When set limits are broken and consequences are given, your child may react strongly. At times, [she] may respond with anger, acting out, and sometimes with depression or withdrawal. Young children may increase angry outbursts in an attempt to test your new behavior plan. Either by acting out or withdrawing, your kids are trying to test your new and improved system of enforcing rules. This shouldn't come as a surprise. Your kids are attempting to find out how serious you are about these rules and consequences. In the heat of giving and following through with a consequence, emotions can really soar.

Today's effective communication skill is aimed at staying CALM while setting limits. See Handout 8C for guidelines.

Use role-play to practice the wrong way and the right way to ease a situation.

Role-Play: Wrong Way/Right Way

The parent comes home to find her child smoking and drinking with a friend. Both parent and child could practice going through the CALM steps but should also be prompted to try an initial reaction they typically would have.

A young child is mad at the parent and picks up a glass vase and throws it on the floor, where it shatters into pieces.

The parent comes home from work and finds the child at home with a friend of the opposite sex when both of them are supposed to be at school.

The parent gets off the phone with the school after having been informed that his child has not been coming to class or has so many missing assignments in a particular class that the child will probably get an F.

TROUBLESHOOTING TIME-OUT WITH YOUNGER CHILDREN

Last week we learned about time-out with younger children, how to use time-out, and some of the ways that time-out can be effective.

QUESTIONS TO ASK PARENTS

➤ Did you use time-out with your child last week? If so, can you describe one time-out situation?

➤ How did the time-out work for your child?

➤ Are there ways you feel the time-out could be improved? If so, how?

Compliment parents for using time-out and whatever they did that was successful. Troubleshoot things that did not go well.

PREDICTING PROBLEMS WITH TIME-OUT

As we discussed last week, anytime you make a change to discipline routines, most children will test the new limits. This often results in an increase in problems for a short time. When you first use time-out, you may see an increase in noncompliance while your children find out whether you really will follow through.

Handout 8D illustrates some common challenges to time-out that parents and children experience.

HOME PRACTICE

Now we're ready to set up home practice. Introduce the rules and consequences that you made earlier during this session for the serious problem behavior you're most concerned about at this time. It's possible that this behavior does not occur on a regular basis or even that it doesn't occur at all right now. But we believe that you, as the expert on your child, know the concerns of the future. You also know that talking with your child now can avoid many problems later on.

Continue to use and track the rules you set last week. Use the tracking form to track how often the rules were broken and the consequences that were given.

When you go home this week, discuss your rules with your child. Remember—be neutral and matter of fact, and avoid criticism.

If your child has been successful with the daily behavior plan, it may be time to move to a weekly reward for completing contracted behaviors. Explain to your child that [she] has been doing well and you think [she] can wait until the end of the week to earn an incentive. You might have to experiment with new incentives that are worth waiting a whole week for. In this case, you can show increased trust and respect for your child's ability to meet your goals. The final stage will be to replace incentives with praise and appreciation for [her] improved behavior. Don't move too quickly to this stage—your child may decide to slip back into old habits.

HOME PRACTICE OUTLINE

1. Introduce rules for serious problem behaviors.

2. Track limits set previously (Handout 6F).

3. Practice time-out (with younger children).

4. Update behavior plans.

Warning Signs to Help Catch Childhood Problem Behavior Early

Aggression and Social Relations

- Wandering or spending time with older peers/siblings

- Fighting or hitting other children

- Lying and/or suspected stealing

- Trouble with basic social skills, such as sharing

- Teacher reporting problems with peers

Inattention/Self-Regulation

- Trouble staying on task at school or home

- Trouble focusing on an activity for extended period of time

- Trouble remembering and following rules

- Emotional outbursts or trouble managing anger

Warning Signs to Help Catch Teen Problem Behavior Early

Substance Use

- Spending time with peers who smoke and use drugs

- Being in unsupervised settings

- Smelling like tobacco, marijuana, or alcohol

- Having notes or any communications about drugs

- Drug paraphernalia

Stealing or Lying

- Having objects without a receipt or a note from a parent

- Being suspected of stealing

- Being suspected of lying

Sexual Involvement

- Spending unsupervised time with boyfriend or girlfriend

- Being out later than an agreed-upon time

- Attending last-minute parties or having dates that are difficult to check

Here is an example of setting consequences and rules for problem behavior.

Teenager

Serious problem behavior: Hanging out with friends who use drugs

Rule: Not allowed at the mall after school or in the evening

Consequence 1: Weekend social privileges removed

Consequence 2: Parent calls friends' parents to discuss problem

Consequence 3: One-hour work chore, such as raking leaves, cleaning stove, vacuuming

Young Child

Serious problem behavior: Hitting sister

Rule: No hitting your sister

Consequence 1: Time-out

Consequence 2: Loss of TV time

Consequence 3: Loss of privilege to play favorite game or with toy for 1 hour

What are some of the problem areas you have to deal with concerning your child?

Serious problem behavior: _____

Rule: _____

Consequence 1: _____

Consequence 2: _____

Consequence 3: _____

From *Everyday Parenting: A Professional's Guide to Building Family Management Skills,* © 2012 by T. J. Dishion, E. A. Stormshak, and K. A. Kavanagh, Champaign, IL: Research Press (www.researchpress.com, 800-519-2707).

- **C**onsider your feelings and thoughts (tense, angry, afraid, shaking)

- **A**ssess whether you are too upset to continue toward a positive outcome at this time.

- **L**eave if you're feeling uncontrollably angry or upset.

- **M**ake a plan to deal with this situation within the next 24 hours.

"We've already tried time-out—it doesn't work."

- Explore previous efforts.
- Look for successes.
- Pinpoint opportunities for improvement.
- Ask questions; look for behavior you can support.
- Get creative, perhaps by renaming time-out or giving time-out to the child's toy.

"There's no place here for a time-out" or "His brother won't leave him alone in time-out."

- Problem-solve, work to tailor time-out to family circumstances.
- Assess pros and cons of different places.
- Consider consequences or incentives for the interfering sibling.

"Time-out isn't severe enough."

- Research has shown that time-out is an effective means to stop or interrupt problem behavior.
- Small consequences are better than large ones for several reasons.
- Think about the importance of consistency with time-out.

Other Possible Challenges

- Parent threatens time-out but does not follow through
- Parent talks with child during time-out
- Parent does not follow up time-out refusal with privilege removal
- Parents disagree about which behaviors receive time-out
- Parent lectures child after time-out
- Child creates messes while in time-out
- Child yells and screams while in time-out

What If My Child Refuses to Go to Time-Out?

Add up to 5 additional minutes, 1 minute at a time.

- When child refuses, stand and wait.
- Say, "That's 1 extra minute."
- With continued refusal, say, "That's 2 extra minutes."
- Add minutes up to 5.

If child still refuses, take away a privilege.

- "That's 6 minutes. Go to time-out now or no cartoons tonight."
- "That's 6 minutes. You can go to time-out now or no video games this evening."
- "That's 6 minutes. You can go to time-out now, or you can't have ice cream this afternoon."

From *Everyday Parenting: A Professional's Guide to Building Family Management Skills,* © 2012 by T. J. Dishion, E. A. Stormshak, and K. A. Kavanagh, Champaign, IL: Research Press (www.researchpress.com, 800-519-2707).

Improving Family Relationships with Negotiation

Overview and Rationale

Conflict is a daily event in every family. How conflict is dealt with in families can have long-term positive or negative effects on all members, and especially on children and adolescents. If families are conflict avoidant, it usually means there is a certain level of unhappiness, fear, anxiety, and resentment that forms the emotional backdrop of daily family life. If conflict leads to escalation and anger, then small problems can grow into large problems, and relationships suffer or end in family breakups or divorce. Problematic family approaches to dealing with conflict have been associated with all forms of major psychopathology, including depression, anxiety, schizophrenia, drug abuse, antisocial behavior, and eating disorders. Helping families address conflict through negotiation can reduce mental health problems among all family members.

Using a proactive and mindful approach and skillful negotiation to address family conflict is vital to building positive family relationships. When handled skillfully, conflict can be a source of growth in family relationships. Successful resolution of conflict renders relationships more resilient and emotional attachments more secure. When family members successfully negotiate conflict, it is safe to deal with problems within the family, and a sense of trust emanates through all interactions.

The major disruptors of skillful resolution of conflict are contempt, defensiveness, criticism, and blame. There are many forms of these behaviors, and ideally the therapist is familiar with each family's style. The Family Check-Up videotaped family interactions are the best source for studying how the family deals with conflict, in what they do, as well as in what they do not do. In particular, a problem-solving task involves the family discussing an area of disagreement that is "hot" for them. Parents' and youths' reports of family conflict may also be used as an assessment tool. However, self-reports of conflict may not be as useful as the videotaped interactions, which provide valuable information about the unique way that conflict disrupts individual families.

The first step in negotiation is the manner in which problems are stated when opening a conflict issue for discussion and negotiation. It may seem paradoxical, but most people bring up conflict situations in a way that seriously compromises the potential for a successful negotiation. For example, "I'm tired of you always whining about going to McDonald's when we go out to eat! You're selfish and never think of other people in the family!" is a direct approach to dealing with conflict, but it is unlikely to lead to a satisfying negotiation for both family members. Alternatively, a parent could calmly say, "Let's talk about how we pick where we go out to eat so we all get a chance to choose." This is a neutral problem statement, and it is vital to healthy negotiation of conflict.

Neutral problem statements can be distinguished from effective requests in that neutral problem statements are used in situations when the parent is open to negotiation. Effective requests are also neutral and do not involve contempt or blame, but they are requests for behavior change that are not negotiable to the parent. Neutral problem statements provide an opening for negotiation and problem solving, and the child's input is welcomed.

Learning the skill of negotiation benefits the youth in several ways. Foremost, youths learn that conflict can be resolved peacefully and that compromise can be satisfying when it leads to improved harmony in close relationships. Second, youths learn to consider another person's perspective when they learn to negotiate and to be more compassionate about others' thoughts and feelings. Parents benefit from successful negotiations in the same way, but they also find that they can relax and share control in some aspects of daily family living and enjoy their child's being more independent and motivated to cooperate.

There is no magic age at which negotiation becomes possible in families. Beginning around age 3, children understand that not everyone sees the world in the same way. Parents can actively structure choices and/or turn-taking in play with peers and siblings. Around age 6 or 7, brainstorming of solutions (see Session 10) is possible. Teaching children negotiation skills early makes considerable sense if it is developmentally appropriate to the participating children. For adolescents, negotiation of conflict and problem solving become critical issues in family life because at this age it is increasingly important to have input into some aspects of family decision making. Conflict is the rule rather than the exception when this does not occur.

SUGGESTED TOOLS

➤ Handout on the don'ts of problem solving

➤ Videotape on bringing up a problem (older or younger versions)

➤ A set of fictitious problems for practice

➤ Questionnaire on negotiation for home experiment

➤ Whiteboard, chalkboard, or large sheets of paper

SESSION OBJECTIVES

➤ Provide overview of negotiation.

➤ Collaboratively identify parents' mistakes in problem solving.

➤ Role-play and rehearse neutral problem statements.

➤ Prepare parents for home practice experiment.

COMMON PITFALLS AND SOLUTIONS

Motivation

An underlying concern that many parents have about negotiation is that some child behavior issues are nonnegotiable. It is helpful for parents to discuss this matter and make a list of issues they would be willing to negotiate up front and a list of those that are expectations or rules. All parents will have some concerns they are willing to negotiate. The other motivational issue is addressing negative emotion in negotiation. It is essential not to lead a family to expect to apply these skills to "hot" topics but to first practice with topics that are not problems or that are less important. One strategy that is helpful when family members push each other's emotional buttons is to problem-solve while sitting back to back in chairs, without directly looking at each other's faces during the interaction. This helps family members focus on what's being said and not be distracted by gestures and body language. Finally, many adults have interpersonal styles they are unaware of that are directly or indirectly critical. The criticism or contempt will leak out when they attempt to use neutral problem statements. For the intervention to be successful, feedback is essential after the neutral problem-solving step is tried at home. It may be advisable to ask parents to hold off and have two sessions to ensure that they can perform the neutral problem statement appropriately.

Tailoring

The child's age and developmental level should be considered when introducing negotiation. In addition, the history of the parents should also be considered. Parents who have limited positive behavior support and/or trouble with limit setting would benefit most from working on these skills rather than on the more advanced parenting skill of negotiation.

Structuring Sessions to Reduce Barriers

Using the handouts will be helpful to structure the discussion of negotiation and especially to encourage the parents to realistically appraise their own style for the purpose of change. It is also helpful to show the videotape about bringing up a problem that is age appropriate.

SETTING THE AGENDA

Greetings. How has the week gone for you in terms of your goal of cooperation with [Chris]?

Today we will talk about negotiation of problem situations with [Chris]. I do think you'll find this topic helpful. These are skills we can use in everyday life not only with our kids but in all close relationships.

I have planned that we would cover the following today (write on a piece of paper, whiteboard, etc., so the parents can see the list):

- Review home practice for last week (if appropriate).

- Review the *don't*s of communication.

- Introduce and rehearse neutral problem statements.

- Introduce the home practice experiment.

Does this seem doable for today? Is there anything else you would like to address? To make sure we get through this and that you feel prepared, I may ask that we put other issues that come up on the back burner to be talked about at the end of our meeting or the next time we meet.

REVIEW OF SESSION 8

To review last session's home practice, let's answer these questions:

- *Did you discuss your expectations and rules concerning the serious problem behavior we talked about last week?*

- *What was the consequence for that rule?*

- *Did you give any consequences for rules that were broken last week? If not, what interfered?*

- *Did you use time-out last week? Did you have any difficulties?*

- *How did it go when you told your child about the plan to set limits?*

- *Did you use any of the consequences last week?*

- *What obstacles prevented you from using a plan or setting limits?*

FAMILY MANAGEMENT SKILL: NEGOTIATION

Objectives

➤ Learn negotiation steps.

➤ Complete the Negotiation Questionnaire on Handout 9A.

➤ Understand negotiation dos and don'ts.

➤ Practice negotiation skills.

As our children get older, we have more opportunities to develop their problem-solving skills. Negotiating with your child is a way to work together to make changes while dealing with problems. At this stage, children need to have more control over their lives. Negotiation gives them a way to bring concerns to you and also to take an active role in managing their own behavior.

Negotiation skills help children focus on solutions rather than on problems. These skills help them think through possible outcomes of their behavior and teach them self-control. Negotiation skills can be learned. Negotiation is not a replacement for discipline. If a situation requires a consequence, a consequence should be given. Negotiation can be a follow-up to discipline to prevent the behavior from becoming a problem in the future.

Five Steps to Negotiation

There are five steps to follow when negotiating:

1. Make neutral problem statements.

2. Generate solutions.

3. Evaluate solutions.

4. Choose a solution.

5. Follow up.

*We will practice the first skill of negotiation, **make a neutral problem statement**, which can often be the most difficult.*

Before we talk more about negotiation, please fill out Handout 9A.

Negotiation Don'ts: Avoiding Common Traps

For the negotiation to go smoothly, there are some common traps to avoid. Let's look at the list of negotiation don'ts *on Handout 9B and identify the ones you have the most difficulty with. These* don'ts *are common traps that families can fall into when trying to change behaviors or in situations in which one or more people may have taken a strong personal interest.*

Keep a list of the don'ts *you find yourself doing. First track your own* don'ts *and then help each other by pointing out when another family member falls into one of the traps.*

Now let's look at the what, when, *and* where *of negotiation on Handout 9C.*

FAMILY COMMUNICATION SKILL: NEUTRAL PROBLEM STATEMENTS

Making neutral problem statements is a key skill that will help you bring up a problem with your child in such a way that [she] is more likely to cooperatively discuss and negotiate a solution.

Now that we've talked about when and where to negotiate and what to avoid, let's talk about the right way to bring up a problem. Successful negotiation must occur in an atmosphere of cooperation. This is done by making neutral problem statements. Staying neutral is easier when the problem is not identified with the person.

Neutral statements cannot guarantee cooperation, but they certainly can help promote it. Making neutral requests is also a good way to teach your children how to communicate with peers.

Remember two things when making neutral problem statements:

First, keep the problem statements brief and specific, leaving no room for misinterpretation.

Second, compliment or recognize the other person's efforts or your own shared responsibility for the problem before you make your neutral statement.

SETTING UP SUCCESSFUL NEGOTIATIONS

The person who states the problem can:

* *Accept part of the responsibility for the problem:* "I know you and I both like to make cookies, and I would appreciate your helping with the cleanup after we make them."

* *Recognize a positive contribution the other person is making related to the problem:* "I appreciate the way you help keep the kitchen cleaned up, and I would appreciate your helping with the cleanup after we make cookies."

* *Give a compliment to the other person:* "You really are a helpful person, and I would appreciate your helping with the cleanup after we make cookies."

* Be **brief**, be **specific**, and use a **neutral** tone of voice.

A list of problems and neutral problem statements for practice with school-age children is provided in Handout 9D. Many of these problems would also be suitable for practice with parents of young adolescents.

Problem Statement: Right Way

Now we're going to practice bringing up a problem the right way. We are not going to try to come up with solutions. It's really important that we bring up the problem in a neutral way so we can encourage cooperation.

Instead of using real problems that you may be having with your child, let's make up some problems. This will make it easier to practice the skill without being distracted by a current hot issue.

Sit back to back. Listen to what your partner is saying. When your partner finishes bringing up the problem, restate what you heard him or her say. Doing this is called "paraphrasing." Your child should be able to paraphrase the problem you bring up. In this way, you can tell that your child understands your view of the problem. Also remember to keep the problem statement neutral, brief, and specific. Before bringing up the problem, remember to give a compliment, take some responsibility, or acknowledge current efforts.

If you are working with one parent, take the role of the child. If you are working with two parents, have the parents turn their chairs back to back, then ask them to practice bringing up the problem. Sitting back to back helps avoid focusing on nonverbal behavior and helps focus on the meaning of the statements.

Parents should practice stating a problem to their child, then take the role of the child and bring up a problem to the parent. All problems during this exercise should be made up and *not* real problems for the parents. Doing it this way avoids any emotional upset or investment in the outcome of the negotiation. Be prepared with a list of made-up problems, although most parents have no difficulty generating them.

Direct the parents to define the problem clearly and specifically. They should make their statements as brief as possible because the other person has to paraphrase. The more that is said, the more room there is for interpretation.

Problem Statement: Wrong Way

Suggest a second role-play for this exercise. Have the parents practice making a problem statement the wrong way, using their favorite *don't*.

Young Children

For some very young children, this exercise may not be developmentally appropriate. However, even very young children benefit from clear discussions of problems and solutions. You can do this exercise with a very young child but keep the discussion brief and direct. Here is an example of a script discussing a problem with a five-year-old:

"I really like the way you play well with your sister. I don't like it when you scream at your sister and use hitting. I want us to work as a family on not screaming and hitting. What do you think?"

HOME PRACTICE

This week, your home practice is to bring up a problem in a neutral way. Remember, you will not try to negotiate a solution yet. That will come next week. Just bring up the problem and arrange a time to talk about solutions next week.

After you bring up the problem with your child, complete the questionnaire on Handout 9E. Next week, we will talk about how you did using the skills we practiced today.

HOME PRACTICE OUTLINE

1. Bring up a problem in a neutral way.

2. Complete Handout 9E.

3. Continue tracking rules and behavior contracts when necessary.

Describe in one or two sentences the most recent problem situation between you and your child.

_____

_____

_____

Is this a typical problem that comes up between the two of you?   ☐ Yes   ☐ No

How angry did this situation make you? *(Circle one number.)*

7	6	5	4	3	2	1
(Very angry)		(Somewhat angry)		(Not angry at all)		

Here is a list of things that often happen in families when they are dealing with problems. Check all that you and your child did while handling this problem.

Parent	Child	Action
☐	☐	Criticized
☐	☐	Lectured
☐	☐	Yelled
☐	☐	Ignored
☐	☐	Discussed
☐	☐	Lost temper
☐	☐	Refused to talk
☐	☐	Threatened
☐	☐	Verbal discipline
☐	☐	Physical discipline
☐	☐	Put down the other
☐	☐	Used sarcasm
☐	☐	Made a joke of it
☐	☐	Asked for more information
☐	☐	Brought up the past
☐	☐	Took away a privilege
☐	☐	Used grounding
☐	☐	Asked a family member to help
☐	☐	Other (*describe*) _____

Describe in one or two sentences how the problem was solved.

_____

_____

_____

From *Everyday Parenting: A Professional's Guide to Building Family Management Skills,* © 2012 by T. J. Dishion, E. A. Stormshak, and K. A. Kavanagh, Champaign, IL: Research Press (www.researchpress.com, 800-519-2707).   **141**

Don't . . .

- **Blame the other person**

Blaming makes the problem the other person's fault. If you say, "It's your fault," then the other person usually becomes defensive and doesn't focus on solving the problem.

- **Defend yourself**

If the other person has stated a problem and you feel responsible or feel you are being blamed, you will feel the need to defend yourself. Let it go or simply say, "I feel like I need to defend myself."

- **Read intentions in another's behavior**

No one is smart enough to know another's thoughts. Family members sometimes think they can do this because they have lived together for a long time, but this is a false assumption. Reading intentions into the behavior of another person keeps that person in a box of old behavior and leads to anger, resentment, and unwillingness to cooperate.

- **Make broad generalizations**

Stick to the topic at hand. If the issue is leaving dishes in the family room, don't add that dishes are also left all over the house, along with shoes, jackets, and books. Small and specific problems are easier to solve.

- **Bring up the past**

The past is often a part of what you don't like now. It's easy to slip into using words such as *always* and *never*. Think of those words as poison when trying to negotiate. This is not the time to bring up that Mom never makes oatmeal for breakfast or that Kylie always leaves her clothes lying on the bathroom floor. These reminders put the person in a box of old behavior, and they don't encourage change.

- **Change the subject**

Stay on track. It is easier to work toward the solution if you stay focused on one topic. If you get sidetracked into related issues, it leads you away from solving the problem.

- **Lecture**

You don't need to give a long explanation or discussion about why you are asking for a change. A simple statement makes it clear. Lectures also lead to many of the other *don'ts*. Using a lot of words lessens people's attention and makes it hard to figure out important information.

- **Put the other person down**

This seems obvious. However, teasing is often a means of humor and closeness in families. It is easy to say something negative about the other under the pretense of teasing.

Don't try to negotiate if you're angry or upset.

From *Everyday Parenting: A Professional's Guide to Building Family Management Skills,* © 2012 by T. J. Dishion, E. A. Stormshak, and K. A. Kavanagh, Champaign, IL: Research Press (www.researchpress.com, 800-519-2707).

What to Negotiate

• What situation do you or your child want to change?

• What daily routines, free time, responsibilities, and rules aren't working? (All are common issues that parents and children negotiate.)

When to Negotiate

• When you have enough free time to discuss a problem.

• When you are not feeling emotional, upset, or stressed.

• When you are not in the middle of the problem.

• When the problem is still manageable.

Negotiation should be done at an unemotional time, not in the middle of the problem. Negotiation should be a calm, thoughtful, and unhurried activity. It should *not* be done at a time when people are upset or stressed. We frequently try to solve problems when we are angry, then we slip into bad habits. As a parent, one of the best ways to stay neutral is to catch problems early, before you have become angry or frustrated. Another way to collect yourself is to make a plan before you approach your child.

Where to Negotiate

• In a neutral spot (e.g., not your child's room or your work area).

• Away from the phone.

• Away from distractions (including other people).

Where to problem-solve depends on each family's situation. We recommend that negotiations occur in a neutral spot in the house, such as the dining room or living room, instead of your child's bedroom. Negotiation should also be done in a place that has the fewest distractions. Don't negotiate in the kitchen because people are usually going in and out. Do negotiate away from the phone and other people's interruptions.

From *Everyday Parenting: A Professional's Guide to Building Family Management Skills*, © 2012 by T. J. Dishion, E. A. Stormshak, and K. A. Kavanagh, Champaign, IL: Research Press (www.researchpress.com, 800-519-2707).

Problem: Morning routine/fighting before school

Neutral Problem Statement: We both like those mornings before school when we get along well. Let's think about ways we can make that happen more often.

Problem: Kids leaving bikes outside where they could be stolen

Neutral Problem Statement: I like that you have fun riding your bikes. Let's talk about how to keep them safe.

Problem: Siblings fighting

Neutral Problem Statement: It's really cool that you guys hang out together so much. Let's talk about how you can get along better.

Problem: Bedtime/going to sleep

Neutral Problem Statement: We both like to have time to read together before bed. Let's think about ways to make sure we have that time.

Problem: Kids fighting in the car

Neutral Problem Statement: Remember last night when we were all laughing in the car? Let's think about ways we can make that happen more often.

Problem: Forgetting to feed pets

Neutral Problem Statement: I love how you hug and play with Kitty. Let's talk about how we can make sure she gets fed every day.

Problem: Homework

Neutral Problem Statement: I know how happy you were when you got that good grade in math. Let's talk about how we can make that happen more often.

Check off what each of you did during your discussion.

What was the problem you used for practice?

_____

_____

	Parent	Child
Initiator		
1. Did you start with …		
a compliment?	☐	☐
recognition?	☐	☐
accepting responsibility?	☐	☐
2. Were you brief and specific?	☐	☐
3. Did you state the problem in a neutral tone of voice?	☐	☐
Partner		
1. Did you repeat to your partner what was said?	☐	☐
2. Were you brief and specific?	☐	☐
3. Did you use a neutral tone of voice?	☐	☐

Choosing Solutions to Family Problems

OVERVIEW AND RATIONALE

Neutrally bringing up a problem is only half the battle. When negotiating conflict in families, the second phase is coming up with possible solutions. This intervention can be challenging to parents because it assumes an attitude of trial and error. That is, the solution to a problem does not necessarily have to be perfect. It's more important that all members have input and, if possible, agree to try the solution for at least a week. As discussed in Session 9, success in this intervention is more likely if parents are willing to negotiate and accept input from the child.

Brainstorming is the core of a positive strategy for coming up with a family solution. Brainstorming involves a time frame in which any family member can suggest a solution without fear of criticism. It is often helpful to purposely generate silly solutions because it promotes humor in resolving conflict, which we know is a valuable strategy for staying engaged in the problem-solving process while releasing tension and reducing negative emotions. In particular, it opens the mind to the idea that there is more than one way to solve a problem, avoiding a common trap in problem solving. Although many parents will understand brainstorming, role-playing the brainstorming process is invaluable.

A frame of reference for this session is building on a success process. Even a failed effort to solve a problem is a success because the family learned from their effort to solve the problem. In this session, we encourage parents to reward effort and not to overly focus on success.

Finally, selecting a solution follows a pros-and-cons approach—systematically going through the list and writing down the pros and cons of each solution, then selecting one solution that has the fewest cons and the most pros. Parent leadership is useful in this phase; there is a balance between taking children's solutions seriously and being the adult who chooses the best possible solution. It is also often possible to compromise and select a solution that is a mixture of two or more family members' ideas.

Clearly, brainstorming should be dramatically simplified for young children age 5 and older. Between ages 2 and 5, simply giving options from which children can choose is a solid foundation for family problem solving in later years. In this session, the parents prepare to practice negotiating with their child and will make a plan to solve a problem.

SUGGESTED TOOLS

> ➤ Handouts on negotiation

> ➤ Age-appropriate videotape of the family attempting to solve a problem or negotiate a solution

> ➤ Fictitious problems for brainstorming

> ➤ Whiteboard, chalkboard, or large sheets of paper

SESSION OBJECTIVES

> ➤ Acknowledge and reward the child's efforts to problem-solve.

> ➤ Give parents an overview of the problem-solving process.

> ➤ Role-play a family negotiation meeting.

> ➤ Prepare the parents for the home practice experiment.

COMMON PITFALLS AND SOLUTIONS

Motivation

Motivation issues similar to those discussed in Session 9 apply to this session as well. The process of brainstorming may be particularly challenging for parents who have high standards and feel the need for considerable control over solutions. Although this dynamic is often difficult to address in terms of the client–therapist relationship, it often reflects the parents' deep concern for getting things right in the family. It is prudent to frequently remind the parents that the solution does not have to be perfect and that engaging the child in the process of negotiation is as important an outcome as success for this week. Let the parents know that involving children in negotiation teaches them to be part of the solution rather than part of the problem. For parents who tend toward criticism, role-playing and modeling a noncritical attitude are key.

Tailoring

Three dimensions are important to consider when tailoring this intervention to best fit a family. First, as discussed earlier, the child's developmental level is highly relevant, and the process should be simplified to appropriately engage the child. Second, the educational background of the family is potentially a factor, and the therapist should define terms such as *brainstorming* or use alternative terms that fit the family's culture and vocabulary. Third, discuss the parents' ability to regulate emotional reactions if they have been a problem in the past. The family problem-solving task during the Family Check-Up offers valuable information for tailoring your work during this session.

Structuring Sessions to Reduce Barriers

This session can be playful and fun if the family is open to humor. If the family is a little more serious in its orientation, setting up the activity as a structured teaching session helps parents engage in role-playing as students and reduces emotional reactions. Following the structure outlined here is important, and avoiding sidetracks is essential. Also, a fictitious problem or a trivial family problem should be used in session practice. When preparing the family for a home practice, the therapist should be actively involved in selecting a problem and should avoid starting off with hot topics. It is better to emphasize using a topic that is manageable so that successful negotiation is achievable. Having an intense conflict in a prescribed negotiation exercise undermines the therapist–client relationship and the parents' sense of self-efficacy.

SETTING THE AGENDA

Greetings. Today we are going to follow up on the negotiation of problems in families. I think you'll find this topic helpful, and some families find the exercises fun! These are skills we can use in everyday life not only with our kids but also with all close relationships.

I have planned that we would cover the following today (write on a piece of paper, whiteboard, etc., so the parents can see the list):

- Review home practice for last week (if appropriate).

- Discuss supporting child's efforts to solve family problems.

- Discuss negotiating solutions to family problems and conflicts.

- Discuss the home practice experiment.

Does this seem doable for today? Is there anything else you would like to address? To make sure we get through this and that you feel prepared, I may ask that we put other issues that come up on the back burner to be talked about at the end of our meeting today or the next time we meet.

REVIEW OF SESSION 9

Last session you were asked to practice making a neutral problem statement to your child. After bringing up the problem, you were asked to fill out Handout 9A, Negotiation Questionnaire, and Handout 9E, the checklist for bringing up a problem.

Discuss information from the questionnaires. Did parents identify certain traps they fall into, such as blaming or lecturing? Review successes with setting limits and behavior plans.

FAMILY MANAGEMENT SKILL: RECOGNIZING EFFORT WHEN CHOOSING SOLUTIONS

Objectives

➤ Learn the skill of recognizing effort in children.

➤ Learn the skills of brainstorming and evaluation.

➤ Practice arriving at a solution.

Recognizing Effort

When your children or adolescents are learning a new skill, recognizing, supporting, praising, and rewarding effort is more important than the outcome—just as it was when you were trying to get them to follow your directions or to complete the steps in your incentive plan. Having children and adolescents participate in brainstorming solutions to problems requires that parents are skilled at recognizing effort rather than recognizing only good ideas.

Right-Way Examples

Problem: Doing the Dishes

Ramon, who is 13 years old, suggests that the family buy a dishwasher, which they do not have, nor can they afford.

> Ramon, I appreciate your speaking up, and it would be good to buy a dishwasher. I'll write down your solution to the problem of doing dishes. Let's have some more solutions, you guys—we will still need someone to load the dishwasher. (Said with a smile and a wink.)

Problem: Arguing About Sitting in the Front Seat of the Car

Briana, who is 5 years old, suggests they sell their car, and then she and her brother, Gene, won't have to argue about who sits in the front seat because they won't have one.

> Yes, Briana, I like the way you said that, and I'll write down the idea that we sell our car. Sometimes I think it's more trouble than it's worth! (Said with a smile.)

Wrong-Way Examples

Problem: Doing the Dishes

> Ramon, why would you say something like that? Buy a dishwasher! It's so frustrating to ask your opinion when all you can do is think about spending money we don't have!

Problem: Arguing About Sitting in the Front Seat of the Car

Briana, selling our car will just make things worse. Think before you give an idea!

Recognizing effort is a key skill in helping two or more people stay on track and in a cooperative frame of mind to negotiate and compromise on a solution to a problem. Let's review the five steps of negotiation:

1. *Make neutral problem statements.*

2. *Generate solutions.*

3. *Evaluate solutions.*

4. *Choose a solution.*

5. *Follow up.*

NEGOTIATION STEPS 2 THROUGH 5

Step 2

Brainstorm by opening your minds and working together. Each person should try to think of as many solutions as possible. Any idea is worth writing down, even those that may seem a little silly or unrealistic. This is where it is very important to recognize a child's efforts to simply contribute to the brainstorming process. Their ideas will give you more choices for solutions. Parents and children should take turns. Try to think of at least three each. You will be surprised at how many solutions even a young child is capable of generating.

Step 3

Evaluate your list of ideas. Practice positive or neutral statements and avoid giving negative feedback about others' ideas. Go back through each idea, one at a time, and list pros and cons. Cross off any ideas that have no pros.

Parents and children should be equal partners in this activity. Encourage your child's ideas and accept [her] evaluations. In the beginning, you will have to guide the process, but your child will become more involved as [she] learns this is a way to make changes.

Step 4

Choose a solution after you have identified the pros and cons of each of your ideas. Choose the solution with the most pros. Sometimes it may be a combination of several ideas. You and your child should accept and agree on the chosen solution. Going through this process helps children think about how their ideas affect themselves and others.

Step 5

Follow up to see how well your solution is working. If you choose a solution that can be tried several times a day, then make a time to check how well it's working. If it's a solution that can be tried only a couple of times a week, then check it in a week.

Try Again!

If you find that your chosen solution isn't working, go back and choose another one or brainstorm a new one. It's hard to know whether a solution will work until you try it out. If it's working, keep it going.

Handout 10B is a Family Negotiation form. An example form is completed (Handout 10A) to show how one family worked together to solve a problem. This week you will have a chance to work on solving a problem and completing the same form.

ROLE-PLAY: NEGOTIATION

Now we're going to use Handout 10B to practice bringing up a problem and coming up with solutions. For this role-play, it's important that we bring up the problem in a neutral way so we can set up the situation for cooperation. Instead of using real problems that you may have with your child, we can choose from some problems I made up. This will make it easier to practice the skill without being distracted by a current hot issue.

Sit back to back and listen to what the other person is saying. When the other person has finished bringing up the problem, tell him or her what you heard. Remember, this is called paraphrasing. Your child should be able to paraphrase the problem you bring up. In this way, you can tell whether your child understands your view of the problem.

Remember to keep the problem statement neutral, brief, and specific. Before bringing up the problem, remember to give a compliment, take some responsibility, or acknowledge your child's current efforts. After making the problem statement, brainstorm and select a solution. Then plan for follow-up.

One parent will play the part of the child, and the other will be the parent. Instruct the parents to follow the negotiation steps. Remind the parents of the *don't*s they want to avoid. Review where and when negotiation should occur.

If you are working with a single parent, you can take the role of the child.

Ask parents how their children will respond to this type of process. Ask parents which behaviors they engage in that may interfere with the negotiation steps.

If time permits, a second role-play for this session would be to have each parent practice solving a problem the wrong way using their favorite *don't*.

NEGOTIATING WITH YOUNG CHILDREN

With younger children, negotiation involves more structure on the parents' part while still allowing the child to have some control over the process and outcome. Young children respond well to negotiating, generating solutions to a problem, and making choices that create a learning context for independence.

Take, for example, bedtime routines, which can be a big problem for many parents of young children. Breaking the routine into steps and outlining those steps for young children can be helpful and promotes success, as well as independence.

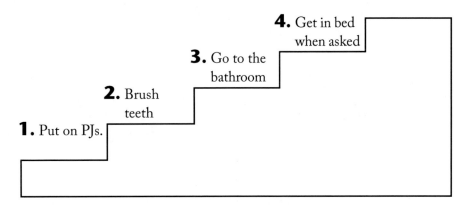

5. Stay in bed

4. Get in bed when asked

3. Go to the bathroom

2. Brush teeth

1. Put on PJs.

Consider the steps depicted here for a successful bedtime routine. One way to negotiate a successful bedtime routine with a young child is to give choices at each step, allowing the young child to have input into the routine, for example, "Do you want to wear red or blue pajamas?" "Do you want to brush your teeth or go to the bathroom first?" "What story would you like to read?"

Choices are one way to negotiate with young children and keep them on track with daily routines.

Parents should practice brainstorming, evaluating, and selecting a solution with their child twice during the week. Procedures used in the session should be followed. Remind parents to:

➤ Sit back to back.

➤ Write down solutions.

➤ Mark each solution with pros and cons.

➤ Keep the list of *don'ts* in mind.

HOME PRACTICE

For this session your home practice is raising a problem and negotiating a solution. Either make up a problem so you and your child can practice the steps or bring up a problem you know will not raise too many emotions.

Complete the Family Negotiation form on Handout 10B and bring it back next week.

After you solve the problem, complete the Negotiation Questionnaire on Handout 9A again. Next week we can talk about how you did using the skills that we practiced during this session.

HOME PRACTICE OUTLINE

1. Bring up a problem and negotiate a solution.

2. Complete a Family Negotiation form.

3. Complete the Negotiation Questionnaire.

4. Rate your child's negotiation skills.

5. Continue any behavior contracts.

6. Continue tracking rules.

Meeting date: _February 10_ Meeting time: _8:30 p.m._   Place of meeting: ___Living room___

Person bringing up the problem: ___Mom___ Person helping solve the problem: ___Allen___

Problem: ___Morning routine___ Was the problem stated in a neutral way? ☑ Yes ☐ No

Ideas to Solve the Problem

1. ___Allen could sleep in and miss 1st period___

   Pros: _____
   Cons: _Allen gets into trouble at school_

2. ___Allen could get up one hour earlier___

   Pros: _____
   Cons: _Allen hates idea_

3. ___Allen could pick out clothes the night before___

   Pros: _Time saving_
   Cons: _____

4. ___Allen could get to shower first___

   Pros: _motivates Allen to get up_
   Cons: _____

5. ___Alen could get up by alarm___

   Pros: _Mom doesn't have to nag_
   Cons: _Allen might go back to sleep_

6. ___If Allen is late, mom goes to work without helping Allen. Mom won't harp
   on Allen and will give only one reminder___
   Pros: _Reduces arguing_
   Cons: _Allen gets into trouble at school_

Solution(s) chosen: ___4, 5, and 6___

Date and time for follow-up meeting: ___next Sunday___

_____   _____
Parent's signature   Child's signature

From *Everyday Parenting: A Professional's Guide to Building Family Management Skills,* © 2012 by T. J. Dishion,
E. A. Stormshak, and K. A. Kavanagh, Champaign, IL: Research Press (www.researchpress.com, 800-519-2707).

Meeting date: _____ Meeting time: _____ Place of meeting: _____

Person bringing up the problem: _____ Person helping solve the problem: _____

Problem: _____ Was the problem stated in a neutral way? ☐ Yes ☐ No

Ideas to Solve the Problem

1. _____

   _____

   Pros: _____

   Cons: _____

2. _____

   _____

   Pros: _____

   Cons: _____

3. _____

   _____

   Pros: _____

   Cons: _____

4. _____

   _____

   Pros: _____

   Cons: _____

5. _____

   _____

   Pros: _____

   Cons: _____

6. _____

   _____

   Pros: _____

   Cons: _____

Solution(s) chosen: _____

Date and time for follow-up meeting: _____

_____   _____

Parent's signature   Child's signature

Proactive Parenting and Planning

Positive Routines That Reduce Stress

OVERVIEW AND RATIONALE

This session is about planning. Having a plan will build family relationships in two fundamental ways. First, parents benefit from understanding the principles behind Everyday Parenting in terms of when to use specific parenting strategies. This level of discussion is clearly best suited for parents who have skills in positive behavior support and healthy limit setting and are actively involved in building positive family relationships. Knowing the principles, they can make a general plan about how to respond to future situations in a way that supports their daughter's or son's growth and competence. The second aspect of planning involves establishing daily family routines that are supportive of effective family management and that promote youths' development.

Parents may be skilled in responding to behavior when it occurs but disorganized in how they approach their day, and many problems may result from this chaos. For example, lack of planning can result in young children having behavior problems during transitions of getting up in the morning and getting ready for school. Teenagers may be bored if they are expected to wait every day in a parent's workplace after school, leading to wandering and potential trouble. A poorly planned routine or schedule may be a barrier to the involvement of children or adolescents in positive activities that are enjoyable and interesting and that promote their skill development and self-regulation.

Positive daily routines that take into account the interests and abilities of the child are understood to be beneficial for youths and to promote their cognitive, social, and emotional development. Helping to make the shopping list and assisting with the shopping can make a mundane activity such as going to the grocery store into a learning experience that increases a child's sense of self-worth. If one looks at children around the world, regardless of a family's amount of financial resources, youths who are involved in the lives of adults in a positive way and have responsibilities such as chores are the most prosocial.

157

This session focuses on this central aspect of proactive parenting. It is general in scope so it can be applied to the diverse needs of families across income, education, and cultural spectra.

SUGGESTED TOOLS

> ➤ Handouts on proactive parenting

> ➤ Whiteboard, chalkboard, or large sheets of paper

SESSION OBJECTIVES

> ➤ Provide an overview of when to use different parenting strategies.

> ➤ Introduce the PLAN strategy for proactive parenting.

> ➤ Role-play gathering information about the youth's interests.

> ➤ Prepare the parents for the home practice experiment.

COMMON PITFALLS AND SOLUTIONS

Motivation

Working on proactive parenting helps parents keep out of the position of reacting to their child's behavior; it is more oriented toward prevention than toward treatment. When faced with behavior problems, emotional distress, and conflict, parents are often intrinsically motivated to practice a skill or an intervention strategy. Proactive parenting, on the other hand, reduces the likelihood of future problems and builds family relationships through positive daily routines. It may be difficult to motivate parents who are not used to this kind of future orientation. However, it is generally true that if they are able to be more proactive for a period of time, parents will experience reduced stress and positive effects on the family and find it deeply rewarding. This experience in and of itself will be helpful for continued mindfulness in family management and daily family routines.

Tailoring

The skill set of proactive parenting is most appropriate to use when parents have a modicum of skill in behavior management and when much of the stress in the family is a result of poor planning of daily routines. If a parent is not skillful in positive behavior support or limit setting, those skills should be supported before addressing proactive parenting. Success in those parenting skills automatically builds more mindfulness in the family. The keys to tailoring this skill set are the family ecology and the developmental level of the child. A parent with monetary resources can hire help to ease the parenting transitions associated with work. Families with less income may need to rely on other resources, such as extended family or reliable friends. Proactive parenting is possible in families of all resource levels, but some families may need to use more creativity as they establish routines that are realistic. The

Family Check-Up is helpful to ensure that this session is applied to the specific circumstances of the family.

Structuring Sessions to Reduce Barriers

The most abstract discussion in this curriculum is the discussion of principles (when to do what). It is helpful for the therapist to come to the session prepared with specific examples that fit the youth's specific behaviors and that are the most appropriate for addressing each parenting skill. Then the information in this session becomes concrete and usable by the family. This applies to proactive planning as well; the therapist should come prepared with specific suggestions tailored to the family, which will begin a discussion on proactive planning of daily routines.

SETTING THE AGENDA

Greetings. How has the week gone for you in terms of your goal of [motivating Chris to complete her homework]? Today we are going to work on supporting you in making plans for the future that will help you and your family by reducing daily stress and improving routines.

I have planned that we would cover the following today (write on a piece of paper, whiteboard, etc., so the parent can see the list):

- Review home practice for last week (if appropriate).

- Discuss when to use which family management skill.

- Make a plan to reduce parenting stress and improve daily routines.

- Discuss discovering your child's interests and using them for routines.

- Discuss the home practice experiment.

Does this seem doable for today? Is there anything else you would like to address? To make sure we get through our agenda and that you feel prepared, I may ask that we put other issues that come up on the back burner to be talked about at the end of our meeting today or the next time we meet.

If you have conducted the family problem-solving sessions with this family, then review Session 10 before moving into the discussion of proactive parenting.

REVIEW OF SESSION 10

Last week our family management skill was recognizing effort when choosing solutions to problems. We talked about family problem solving and, in particular, coming up with solutions that you should try for only one week. Are there any questions about the information presented last session?

Your home practice last session was to solve a problem with your child. After bringing up the problem and working on a solution, you were going to complete the Negotiation Questionnaire. Let's start with your telling me the problem you decided on, how it was brought up, if it was solved, and how your child reacted to the negotiation process. Did you have any problems coming up with a mutually agreeable solution? With younger children, you were going to give choices to shape behavior. How did this plan work with your younger child?

Discuss information from the Negotiation Questionnaire. Ask parents to identify traps they fell into, such as blaming or lecturing. Give parents an opportunity to talk about current behavior contracts. Find solutions to difficulties they may be having and encourage them to continue their efforts. Quickly review successes at setting limits.

BEHAVIOR CONTRACTING, SETTING LIMITS, AND NEGOTIATION

The skills you have learned and practiced here and at home, if continued, will result in positive communication in your relationship with your child. It's important to try to keep up an equal measure of encouragement and limit setting, combined with continued involvement and supervision of the child's behavior outside the home.

Make time for discussions with your teen and playtime with your young child. Many families find that a weekly time for family meetings is also productive for increasing communication.

The skills you have learned may take a little more time to feel natural, but the more often skills are practiced, the more they'll become a part of the family routine. The skills that tend to fall away most easily are daily encouragement and setting up behavior plans to encourage changes in behavior. All of us have to work hard to focus on positive behaviors because negative behaviors catch our attention more easily.

In reality, many of the skills you've learned serve the same purpose. For example, the behavior-change plans, monitoring, setting limits, and negotiation skills do the same thing: guide our children's behavior. The challenge is to decide when to use which method. Although there is no simple formula for making those decisions, I can offer some suggestions. To decide what to do, ask yourself these questions:

- *What is the problem?*

- *Have I defined the problem (pinpointing)?*

- *Have I identified a positive goal?*

- *Have I tracked the behavior?*

- *What are the ABCs (antecedents, behavior, consequences) of this behavior?*

If you have defined and tracked the behavior, you are ready to decide which method to use. If you have not defined or tracked the behavior, do not begin until you have. When you have completed the preliminary steps, continue.

Review the questions on Handout 11A to decide which problem-solving skill to use.

*This week our family management skill is called **proactive parenting**, and our communication skill is focused on talking with your child to gather information. We will talk about ways to be a proactive parent and about effective ways to ask your child questions and gather information, which is part of building a strong relationship between you and your child.*

FAMILY MANAGEMENT SKILL: BEING A PROACTIVE PARENT AND STOPPING PROBLEMS BEFORE THEY OCCUR

Continue:

By being proactive, you can actually prevent problem behaviors and emotional upset in your children. Little things such as telling your child ahead of time about transitions or changes can help [her] prepare for a stressful situation. Examples:

- *"In five minutes, we are going to leave, and you will need to put away your toys."*

- *"This weekend, we are going camping, so don't make any plans with Nancy to play."*

- *"If your brother comes home this weekend, you will need to stay home Friday night."*

Parents who can anticipate and prevent problem behavior by being proactive use a more positive attitude and reward the behavior they want to see instead. Children experience their proactive parents as more positive, supportive, confident, and in control.

Proactive parenting is helpful for children and adolescents when choices are given so children can contribute to solutions for how to deal with the future event:

- *"Do you want to start picking up your toys now, or would you like to wait two minutes?"*

- *"Would you like to make a play date with Nancy this Thursday or next week after we get back?"*

- *"Do you want to call your brother and see if he has any plans on Friday night?"*

Proactive parenting has a stronger, more positive influence on children's development of positive behaviors than does limit setting or other parenting strategies. It functions to teach children appropriate behavior through structuring, provides a predictable learning environment, and helps children with their emotional regulation.

What Is Proactive Parenting?

The process of proactive parenting can be summarized by the acronym PLAN, identified below and explained on Handout 11B. The main ideas behind proactive structuring are presented in that handout, which will help you make a PLAN:

P = **P**ay attention and identify troublesome situations for your child.

L = **L**ook realistically at your child's abilities in that situation.

A = **A**djust difficult activities to maximize success and minimize negative emotions.

N = **N**ever forget to prompt, suggest, and reward success!

Using proactive structuring requires some preparation by parents. Here are some guidelines for making successful use of proactive parenting:

- *New situations: Pay particular attention when a situation is new to the child or when a new problem behavior occurs.*

- *Boredom: Anticipate when the child may become bored and frustrated, and take steps to prevent trouble before it arises.*

- *Difficult tasks: Ease the child through a difficult task or situation by giving helpful information about what is expected or by offering reasons or incentives before a task starts and/or before the child becomes frustrated.*

- *Structure child's time and activities: Use scaffolding, or structuring, of the child's time and activities (e.g., from short to long, from fast to slow, from easy to more difficult) to maintain [her] interest.*

- *Allow child to help: By suggesting appropriate activities to the child, allow [her] to help with the task, engage in an activity [she] can then assume independently, and help [her] only as much as needed.*

Examples of Proactive Parenting

Proactive Parenting with a Young Child: Grocery Store

Many parents have difficulty with their young children in the grocery store. The ideal proactive solution is to schedule a time to do grocery shopping without your children. However, that is not always possible. A proactive approach would be the following:

- *While you are still in the car, tell children what is expected of them in the grocery store ("no fighting; stay in the cart").*

- *Keep shopping trips brief.*

- *Tell children they will earn a reward for good behavior in the store (pick out their favorite cookies, etc.).*

- *Make sure to give children their reward if they earn it and praise success along the way.*

Proactive Parenting with an Adolescent: Computer Time

Many parents struggle with their teens over computer use. Parents want to limit time and monitor websites their teens visit, and teens want full access to the computer. Try this proactive approach to computer use with your teen:

- *Keep computers in a public area of the household, such as the kitchen or TV room. Do not have computers in bedrooms.*

- *Computer time is a privilege. Let your teen earn computer time by completing homework, doing chores, and so forth.*

- *Limit time to a specified amount each day that you work out in advance with your teen.*

- *Monitor what websites your teen uses by sitting down with [her] at the computer on occasion and talking about [her] computer use.*

Handout 11C provides a list of possible trouble spots that many families experience with their children. Check the trouble spots for your family and consider whether these are changes that you want to work on.

TROUBLESHOOTING: PROACTIVE PARENTING STRATEGIES

Effective use of proactive parenting strategies requires a commitment to thinking differently. Ongoing review, debriefing, and troubleshooting strengthen a parent's ability to use this way of thinking and planning to prevent the occurrence of misbehavior.

Identify what is working well, identify any problem areas, such as what is interfering with successful implementation, and make adjustments accordingly. Parents can use a questioning process to help evaluate ways to use their teaching skills to promote their children's success. Parents should ask themselves:

➤ Did I identify the correct behavior to prevent?

➤ Did I correctly identify the situation that results in the behavior I want to avoid?

➤ Did I look well enough at all the times the behavior is occurring?

➤ Did I respond in one or more of the following ways to prevent the behavior from occurring?

  - Explain what will happen next

  - Give some choices

- Give warnings when activity will begin or end

- Distract

- Redirect

- Eliminate the object, person, or activity functioning as the trigger **before** the child arrives

- Suggest to the child (or engage the child in) an alternate, interesting situation

➤ Did I notice what happened as the result of the changes in my behavior?

FAMILY COMMUNICATION SKILL: TALKING WITH YOUR CHILD OR ADOLESCENT AND GATHERING INFORMATION

Many parents struggle to talk with their child so they can figure out what their child is thinking or feeling about situations. For example, consider this scenario, which is common among many parents:

Lucy, a second grader, came home from school very upset on Wednesday. Her mother asked her what was wrong, and Lucy simply stated "nothing" and pouted in her room for the rest of the afternoon. Later that night, Lucy refused to do her homework. She became angry when her mother asked her to get her homework done before having a snack and started yelling and screaming. Her mother asked her again, "Is this about what happened at school?" Lucy screamed, "Nothing happened at school, so stop asking!"

Many parents have had a similar frustrating interaction with their child when they are quite sure the child had a negative experience or something happened at school, but they cannot seem to get the information about this incident from their child.

Handout 11D is a set of skills for gathering information from young children and adolescents. These tools are useful when children are too young to tell the whole story or they are too upset. These tools are also helpful with adolescents who are reluctant to tell their parents about their day.

HOME PRACTICE

Explain the home practice:

This week, gather information from your child about [her] day. Use some of the skills we have discussed earlier and see what new information you can learn from your child.

Using Handout 11C, identify an area you can change using proactive parenting. Develop a PLAN for changing this problem and implement the plan this week.

You have now learned many of the skills you will need to form a healthy, positive relationship with your child. The best way to keep up a healthy re-

lationship with your child is to continue to use these skills regularly. Every family will have setbacks, and each child will respond differently to these new parenting strategies. If you keep up these skills with your child, you will continue to help your child grow into a successful adult.

Am I willing to negotiate a
solution to this problem?

If yes, use negotiation skill. If
no, continue to the next option.

Am I willing to create a
behavior-change plan to solve
this problem?

If yes, use incentive contracts. If
no, continue to next option.

Am I willing to set limits on this
behavior?

If no, begin again. Talk to a
professional or a supportive
friend.

From *Everyday Parenting: A Professional's Guide to Building Family Management Skills,* © 2012 by T. J. Dishion,
E. A. Stormshak, and K. A. Kavanagh, Champaign, IL: Research Press (www.researchpress.com, 800-519-2707).

P = **P**ay attention and identify troublesome situations for your child.

L = **L**ook realistically at your child's abilities in that situation.

A = **A**djust difficult activities to maximize success and minimize negative emotions.

N = **N**ever forget to prompt, suggest, and reward success!

Parenting Practices That Are Proactive

• Explain what will happen next.

• Give some choices.

• Give warnings when activity will begin or end.

• Distract child with alternative activity or toy.

• Redirect child or adolescent with alternative activity.

• Eliminate "triggers" that may create negative emotional reactions.

• Teach or suggest to the child a coping skill.

Examples

Your 4-year-old refuses to get dressed in the morning and watches TV instead.

P = What is the problem? (Getting dressed in the morning.)

L = Can your child dress himself? (Yes, if you lay his clothes out for him.)

A = Adjust for success. (Lay out clothes; keep the TV off until he's dressed.)

N = Don't forget to tell him what a good job he did! (And let him watch his TV show.)

Your 12-year-old is not doing homework but is watching TV, playing on the computer, and listening to music at the same time!

P = **What is the problem?** (Not completing homework.)

L = **For how long can your child do homework without distractions?** (30 minutes)

A = **Adjust for success.** (Create a place for doing homework separate from distractions. Make 15 minutes of computer use or listening to music contingent on doing 30 minutes of homework.)

N = **Don't forget to tell her what a good job she did!** (Acknowledge her efforts and notice when she is independently working on homework.)

Make a PLAN of Your Own

P = _____

L = _____

A = _____

N = _____

From *Everyday Parenting: A Professional's Guide to Building Family Management Skills,* © 2012 by T. J. Dishion, E. A. Stormshak, and K. A. Kavanagh, Champaign, IL: Research Press (www.researchpress.com, 800-519-2707).

Consider the following list of trouble spots for many children. Do any of the following apply to you and your child? If so, use a checkmark to indicate trouble spots and to indicate which of them you would like to change using proactive parenting.

	Trouble spot?	Want to work on it?
Bedtime	☐	☐
Going shopping	☐	☐
After school/homework	☐	☐
Computer usage	☐	☐
Getting ready to go out	☐	☐
Bath time	☐	☐
Visiting friends	☐	☐
Having guests at the house	☐	☐
While I'm doing chores	☐	☐
While I'm on the phone	☐	☐
On car trips	☐	☐
While I'm making meals	☐	☐
After I go to bed	☐	☐
When I am at work	☐	☐
Having friends at the house	☐	☐
Other (*Specify:* _____)	☐	☐

Give children some time to settle in and relax. Spend some time eating a snack with your child, watching TV, or just relaxing while you pay attention to your child and listen.

Start by using reflective listening statements such as the following:

• Tell me about the play you've been practicing.

• What do you like to do at recess?

• Wow, I can see that you are excited; tell me why.

Young children respond well to closed-ended questions about their day. They have trouble answering a question such as "How was your day?" It is too vague and will usually result in a brief answer, such as "fine." Consider the following examples:

• Whom did you eat lunch with?

• Did you have PE today?

• Whom did you play with on the playground?

• Did you go on the swing?

• Was your friend Cameron on the bus?

Older children respond well to open-ended yet direct questions such as the following:

• How was math class today?

• Seems like you enjoy track; tell me about it!

• Did you see your friend John today at school? How did that go?

• What did you do during your breaks today at school?

Giving choices is another way to gather information from children. Questions that do not elicit a choice (e.g., "Are you mad?") can often elicit defensiveness in a child and limit discussion. Consider the following examples:

• Would you say you are more mad or sad?

• If 10 is really mad, and 1 is not mad at all, how mad are you?

Shared Family Routines

Communication Skills That Promote
Engagement and Enjoyment

OVERVIEW AND RATIONALE

Building a relationship with a child or adolescent takes time and involves skillful engagement in the routines of family life that occur daily, weekly, monthly, and yearly. For example, shopping for groceries, visiting friends, family recreational activities, sports, and even going to the dump can be made into a parent–child adventure. Family relationships unfold in the context of routine activities involving parents and youths. Positive family routines with children and adolescents build trust and communication. Trust is built by the adult's reliably showing up and carrying out the routine as promised. Communication is strengthened by unobtrusive support and interest in discussions that are appealing for the adult and child. Strong family relationships are a compass that will help the family navigate inevitable storms, such as marital problems, the transition from childhood to adolescence, and health and work problems.

There are two major scenarios in which the adult–child relationship may require attention and may benefit from a shared family routine intervention. In the first, the relationship with a parent is weak because of some kind of disruption, and the parent has been absent physically or psychologically. This may stem from drug and alcohol addiction; mental health problems, such as depression; trauma in the family, such as divorce; unrelenting work schedules that disrupt family life; or a parent who struggles with close relationships with his or her children because of his or her own history. The second and more common scenario is the reconstituted stepparent situation in which a new parent who does not have an existing relationship with the children is inserted into a family situation. The stepparent's relationship with a child can become more challenging if the child perceives that the new parent was involved in the divorce or if the new stepparent assumes a parenting role too quickly. A new relationship may seem like a very positive development in the life of a parent, but it is likely to be experienced very differently by the children involved. In this sense, a new and sudden marriage can create a schism in family communication and mutual understanding that requires attention, planning, and skill to overcome. Rebuilding family relationships with healthy boundaries is the first step to recovery in new stepparent families.

This session builds on the skills covered in all the other sessions in the Everyday Parenting curriculum. This session emphasizes communication skills that open the door to communication, mostly by engaging the child or adolescent. Young children can be engaged by techniques often referred to as *child-directed play*. This involves leaving some room in the day (even 5 minutes) in which the parent follows the lead of the child when spending time together. This same skill evolves as children grow into school age, when they may be given choices and input into how routine activities are carried out. Finally, by adolescence, simply spending time and creating an atmosphere of voluntary communication can do wonders when families approach and discuss sensitive topics, such as drug use, sexual behavior, and/or relationship choices. Figure 10 provides an overview of the parents' role in developing positive communication with a child or adolescent.

Proficient communication with a child is one of the most valuable skills that a parent can offer the relationship. With young children, this skill comes with talking, playing, and spending time together in activities. The key for younger children is for a parent to spend dedicated time with them, giving them their full attention. With older children and adolescents, a parent's style of communication can be the key to building a relationship. To develop a strong relationship with a child or adolescent, it is essential that parents are able to talk about sensitive issues that are important to both of them. One way that a parent closes the door to communication is by intruding into the life of the adolescent, asking questions about sensitive topics without engaging the youth in the conversation. Time spent with a child or adolescent goes a long way toward gaining an understanding of the right time to have a sensitive discussion. Activities such as driving a son or daughter to a sporting event with friends and listening to their conversation provides rich information about how they are experiencing their world and perhaps indicates aspects of the youth's life in which adult support is needed.

The Family Check-Up provides a venue for assessment of parent communication and listening skills, as well as feedback. The family assessment session can be used to provide information to the therapist and parents about listening skills and to stimulate a discussion of sensitive topics (e.g., substance use). While practicing the communication skills, it is suggested that parents begin with benign topics and leave more sensitive issues, such as divorce or other acute stressors, until the skill matures (following the lead of the child or adolescent).

FIGURE 10 **A parent's role in developing good communication and a positive parent–child relationship.**

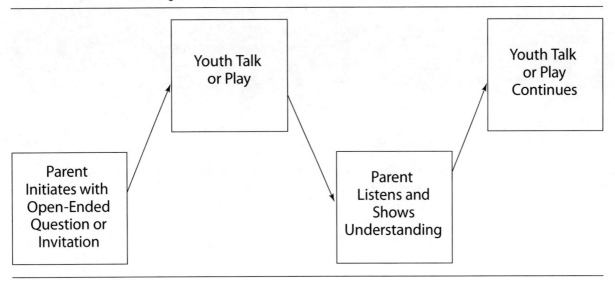

SUGGESTED TOOLS

➤ Videotaped examples of parent using communication and listening skills with a child

➤ Handouts on active listening and family communication profile

➤ Shared Family Routine handout

➤ Whiteboard, chalkboard, or large sheets of paper

SESSION OBJECTIVES

➤ Role-play with parents open-ended questions and active listening skills.

➤ Support the parents' skills in attending to their child.

➤ Help parents identify their thoughts and feelings that act as barriers to communication and listening.

➤ Prepare parents for a successful interaction with their child using communication and listening skills.

COMMON PITFALLS AND SOLUTIONS

Motivation

Many of the barriers to communication and listening are related to parents' own communication and listening skills and patterns. For example, a parent who is depressed and tired is less able to structure times to talk directly with his or her children. Parents who have several children and lead more stressful lives are also less likely to be able to find time to talk with each child. Adapting the home practice and role-plays to accommodate these issues helps these parents achieve success. In some situations, parents may be too eager or desperate to form a relationship with a child, especially in stepparent families. From a stepparent's perspective, the child may "hold the cards" as to whether the adult relationship will succeed. It is helpful to address these motivation issues up front, to normalize the situation, and to suggest that starting small and being persistent is better than overwhelming the child with unwelcomed overtures.

Tailoring

The child's age and developmental level must be seriously considered when tailoring communication and listening skills. With younger children, tailoring involves setting aside time to focus exclusively on the child. With older children, it may involve more advanced skills, such as problem solving and negotiation. Ideally, each parent will have a plan for communication with each child in the family, and the plan should be based on the child's developmental level. The plan also may vary based on the behavior of the child. Some children are talkative and easy to communicate with, whereas others are withdrawn and shy. Attention should be paid to the temperament of the child and to the contextual stressors of the parent that may inhibit communication. While parents complete the exercises, emphasize the importance of knowing about the child's style and trying to work with that style. It's probably most difficult to communicate with a child who doesn't talk a lot. After acknowledging this, ask the parents to brainstorm strategies for promoting communication (e.g., humor, working together, watching and talking about a TV show together, playing a game). Tailoring is critical to forming appropriate expectations for adult efforts and to helping parents feel confident their efforts will work.

Structuring Sessions to Reduce Barriers

First, address barriers related to context and stress in the parents' lives. Many parents simply state that they do not have time to spend talking to their children. Help the parent complete the Shared Family Routine handout as a process for addressing barriers. It is vital for the parents to thoroughly discuss these barriers and problem-solve with the therapist. These parents should be encouraged to start small, finding even 5 minutes a day to practice skills with each child. Role-plays with parents, and with older children and parents, may facilitate this process. Once parents have made time, they will find that communicating with their children is usually rewarding and therefore easier to continue in the future.

SETTING THE AGENDA

Good to see you again. Last session we talked about the PLAN approach to proactive parenting. Today I'd like to spend some time with you going over that experience and troubleshooting any problems that came up. Before we begin, has anything happened since the last time we met that I should know about before we move forward?

If anything has happened that would affect parents' skill development during the session, it should be briefly addressed, and they should be asked if they are ready to continue the work started in the previous session.

I have planned that we would cover the following today (write on a piece of paper, whiteboard, etc., so the parents can see the list):

- Review PLAN and proactive parenting, troubleshooting.

- Complete a family communication profile.

- Complete the Shared Family Routine exercise.

- Role-play open-ended questions and active listening skills.

- Discuss the home practice experiment.

Does this seem doable for today? Is there anything else you would like to address?

Be responsive to the parents' concerns, or tailor the list by adding items such as *two parents with different communication styles* if you want to deal with a family dynamic in which only one parent has the skills to communicate effectively.

REVIEW OF SESSION 11

Let's take a minute to review what we've learned so far before talking about how your week went. Last session, we focused on the PLAN approach to proactive parenting. We also learned about ways to gather information from your child and build your relationship through talking, listening, and questioning.

We learned a great deal about how family stress and problem behavior could be reduced by (1) paying attention and identifying your child's problem situations, (2) looking realistically at your child's skill level, (3) actively prompting or suggesting positive behavior and giving choices, and (4) never forgetting to reward and praise your child's success.

Discuss the parents' proactive parenting strategies during the past week. Give parents the opportunity to talk about ways they used proactive parenting with their child. Discuss any problems or barriers parents may have had to coming up with a proactive plan (e.g., busy schedules, not enough time).

QUESTIONS TO ASK PARENTS ABOUT PROACTIVE PARENTING

➤ What situations did you find to be most troublesome?

➤ How did you change or restructure the situation?

➤ Was it successful?

➤ How would you approach the situation proactively in the future?

➤ How did proactive parenting differ for the different ages of your children?

FAMILY COMMUNICATION SKILL: COMMUNICATION THAT ENHANCES FAMILY RELATIONSHIPS

Objectives

➤ Identify family communication profile

➤ Learn and practice open-ended questions and active listening skills

The Family Communication Profile helps parents make a self-assessment of their family's communication style.

Briefly identify the topics that you have and haven't talked about with your child. What topics are important to discuss with your children?

It is necessary for your children to challenge your thinking and your behavior from time to time if they are going to adopt your values and obey your rules when you are not present. For example, if you preach that smoking is harmful and you smoke, your [daughter] may ask why you are doing something that is bad for your health. If you model social relationships that are prosocial and healthy, your child will likely have similar friendships at school. If a family value is honesty, yet one of the adults is observed to be dishonest in some relationships, then children and especially adolescents will doubt the value.

Promoting Good Communication

*The first step in promoting good communication between you and your child is to **clarify** what you want to teach your child about a particular subject. It's hard to communicate clearly about topics that are personally confusing or that elicit strong emotions (e.g., honesty, sexual behavior, or divorce). You also have to be willing to hear information that may be hard to listen to. If you find out your child has stolen something or has been skipping school, then you need to do something about it.*

We have emphasized the role of parents as a child's main resource for learning and decision making. To be most effective, you need to stay involved. One way to do this is by setting aside time to talk in the context of shared family routines, when talking is not the main focus.

Talking can happen in a variety of settings—in the car, doing errands and chores together, and sometimes during dinner. Some families have a set time and place for communication (i.e., family meetings). A word of caution: Parents often try to do other things while communicating with their children. For instance, listening often happens in the middle of cooking, working, doing something with another child, or watching TV. Then we ask, "Why don't our kids talk to us?" If we encourage our children to talk with us, we need to show them we're interested in what they're saying.

Let's take a survey of your family's communication style and what kinds of communicators your children are. You could have a Nonstop Nick, who talks from the minute he gets up in the morning. It's hard to know when to listen to him. On the other hand, you could have a Silent Sarah, who can barely get out a one-word response when you ask a question.

Children differ widely in their communication styles and may respond differently depending on the day, the place, and who is present. Let's look at Handout 12A, the Family Communication Profile.

Shared Family Routines

Now let's see about opportunities you have to talk, or communicate, with your child. Shared family routines are events that occur regularly and offer an opportunity for you and your child to choose each of your roles in the activity. For example, on a family outing, both the parent and child can select one fun activity during the outing. When identifying family routines on the handout, make sure they are routines that are realistic and ones that your child would be able to give constructive input into even though you are the leader. Note that some routines occur daily, others weekly, monthly, or even yearly. Let's focus now on the daily and weekly routines. The same idea holds for those that don't occur so often.

Handout 12B gives some examples of shared family routines. Please fill out Handout 12C, then we'll talk about it when you have finished.

OPEN-ENDED QUESTIONS AND INVITATIONS: THE START-UP PHASE

The same skills that apply to neutral problem statements apply to open-ended questions. Open-ended questions are designed to start a conversation and are open to any response from the child. Some examples of open-ended questions include:

- *"Hey, I have some time off on Saturday—anything you want to do?"*

- *"It seems like a long time since we took a bus ride, so what do you think about doing that sometime?"*

- *"Would you like to watch some movies tonight? You pick one and I'll pick one."*

- *"How did school go today? I heard that you came home upset."*

On the other hand, here are some questions that are not open ended:

- *"I have from 2 to 4 off this Saturday afternoon. Let's go down to the racetrack."*

- *"I'm going to take the bus to the city tomorrow and I want you to go with me."*

- *"We are going to watch movies tonight, but I don't want you to watch anything violent."*

- *"I heard you were upset today when you came home from school. Did you screw up again?"*

ACTIVE LISTENING PHASE: KEEP THE WHEELS ROLLING

Make sure it's a good time to focus on listening and that you're not doing something else, such as cooking, reading, watching TV, or working on the computer.

Do...

- *Show understanding.*

- *Summarize what your child said.*

- *Practice patience.*

- *Emphasize positive behaviors and choices.*

- *Repeat what your child said; ask if you understood correctly what was said.*

- *Ask closed-ended, direct questions (e.g., "Whom did you eat lunch with today?" vs. "What did you do at school today?").*

Don't...

- *Interrupt or interpret*

- *Accuse*

- *Think about intentions*

- *Blame or criticize*

- *Give advice*

CREATE A FOUNDATION FOR COMMUNICATION

Some younger children are not yet able to focus on talking and communicating for long periods of time. For younger children, it is important to set aside time each day for listening and communicating, but it may occur in the context of playtime or story time. Focusing on your child for at least 10 minutes a day will improve your relationship and create a foundation for later listening and communication. Asking a younger child specific questions rather than vague, open-ended questions may also facilitate communication. For example, "Whom did you sit next to at lunch?" is better than "How was lunch today?"

ROLE-PLAY: COMMUNICATION SESSIONS

The role-play is designed to help parents practice skills. Have parents practice listening skills with you or with each other. First, have them listen to a typical situation and practice listening and asking questions. Then give parents a more serious or emotional situation. The goal of this role-play is for the parents to (1) practice patience, (2) show understanding, and (3) emphasize success. In the role-play, the parent playing the child will be given a scenario. The parent in the role-play will be allowed to respond only with items from the statements listed below. The parent needs to choose when to show patience, when to use a phrase of understanding, and when to emphasize success.

Patience	Understanding	Success
Say nothing.	"That must have been hard."	"You did great!"
Nod head.	"I would have felt that way."	"Way to go!"
"Uh-huh."	"That was difficult."	"That's super!"
"Yes."	"I bet that felt awkward."	"Wow!"

Scenarios for School-Age Children

Listening Script 1: Jack

Background: Jack is hyperactive and has a hard time controlling his behavior when playing with other kids.

Story: Today, Jack was playing tag with some other boys on the playground. One of the boys ran into the play structure and blamed Jack. The teacher on duty saw the whole thing and brought both boys inside to discuss what had happened. She said that it was an accident and that Jack had not caused the other boy to get hurt, but she did notify Jack's parents.

Scene: Jack is with his dad, driving to pick up a package at the post office.

Listening Script 2: Abby

Background: Abby is a sensitive girl who had a very close relationship with her father until he remarried. She is jealous of the attention that he pays to her stepmom. She has started stealing from other kids.

Story: Abby was playing at her friend Maria's house. Abby really liked one of Maria's little action figures and spent a lot of time playing with it. When it was time to go home she put it back in the wrong spot, and Maria thought she had taken it. However, Maria's mom had found that it was just misplaced.

Scene: Maria is making desserts for the family dinner on Sunday, and she is talking with her grandmother, who is her primary caregiver.

Scenarios for Adolescents

Listening Script 1: Ben

Background: Ben has been hanging around with a new friend, Jake. His parents are concerned about who he is hanging out with and what the boys are doing. The parents haven't heard much about Ben's new friend and would like to know more.

Story: Ben arrives home from school later than usual. He says he was at the mall with Jake, who wanted him to shoplift a CD from the music store. Ben is not supposed to go to the mall without permission. He decided that stealing a CD was a bad idea. He also told Jake that he would stop hanging out with him if he tried to talk him into doing illegal things. Jake called Ben a "chicken" and Ben left, deciding that he does not need friends like Jake.

Scene: Mom, Dad, and Ben are having dinner together. Dad starts the conversation by asking him how his day went with Jake.

Ben: "Well … I went to the mall."

Listening Script 2: Tanya

Setup: Tanya is an early-maturing middle school student whose parents are concerned about her involvement with boys and possible sexual behavior.

Scenario: Today at school, the boy who has been calling Tanya put his arm around her when they were walking down the hall. She asked him politely to remove his arm, but he acted as if she was joking. The principal happened to see them and called them into her office to talk about showing affection at school. Tanya later asked the boy not to call her anymore and told him she never wants to see him again.

Scene: Tanya is delivering papers with her mother and seems upset. Mom asks, "What happened at school today?"

HOME PRACTICE

For an Older Child

This time for home practice, you're going to need your child's help. I'd like you to set up a time during the week that you can practice your active listening skills with [Chris]. You need to do this only once, but you can do it more often if you want.

For a neutral situation, ask your child to talk with you about [her] day at school. You should ask [her] at the end if she thought you were listening and what specifically you did that made [her] feel you were listening.

For older children, I'd like you to have them talk about a more sensitive is-sue such as friends [she] likes that you don't approve of, drug use, or sexual behavior. Tell [her] your assignment is to find out what [she's] thinking. This isn't a session to decide or change anything. You'll offer no opinions unless your child asks for one.

Again, ask your child for feedback. Did [she] feel you listened, based on what you did?

For a Younger Child

For this home practice, set up a time each day to play with your child. During this time, let your child take the lead on games and activities [she] would like to play, and you will follow along. This is called "child-directed play." Playing with your young child is an important way for you to en-hance your positive relationship with your child. It is also how children learn to express emotions, try out roles, and communicate thoughts and feelings about their world.

Refer to these guidelines when playing with your young child this week.

- *Follow the child's lead by doing what your child wants to do during play and by summarizing what your child says and does (e.g., "You are making a block tower").*

- *Watch carefully and sit next to your child.*

- *Ignore inappropriate behaviors unless they are dangerous.*

- *Give the child time to think and explore.*

- *Listen to the child's play and follow along.*

- *Do not give commands or try to structure the play.*

- *Do not use the time to teach (such as ABCs, etc.).*

- *Use lots of praise and support ("Great job!").*

- *Let your child know you enjoyed spending this time with [her].*

HOME PRACTICE OUTLINE

1. Continue behavior plan if necessary.

2. Monitor and enforce limits when necessary.

3. Practice listening with older child and playing with younger child.

4. Have older children fill out the questionnaire on Handout 12D.

How would you describe your communication style?

_____

_____

How would you describe your child's communication style?

_____

_____

Do you have a regular time and place to talk?

_____

_____

What are the times you are most available?

_____

_____

Where and when is your child most comfortable talking (e.g., riding in the car, at bedtime)?

_____

_____

What is something you do that promotes good communication?

_____

_____

What is something you do that interferes with your listening or talking with your child?

_____

_____

What is something your child does that interferes with your ability to listen or talk with him or her?

_____

_____

Shared Family Routine Form (Completed Example)

Frequency	Shared routine	Child's input (picks one element or activity)	Parent's input (picks one element or activity)
Daily	Walking dog Cooking dinner	Chooses route Chooses to chop veggies	Chooses time to go Chooses main dish
Weekly	Go downtown Sporting event	Chooses favorite store Chooses what to wear (team colors)	Chooses the day Chooses the event
Monthly	Trip to the ocean Bike ride or hike	Chooses state park Chooses the route/place	Chooses duration Chooses the weekend
Yearly	1-week vacation	Chooses to see the aquarium	Chooses the location to visit

From *Everyday Parenting: A Professional's Guide to Building Family Management Skills*, © 2012 by T. J. Dishion, E. A. Stormshak, and K. A. Kavanagh, Champaign, IL: Research Press (www.researchpress.com, 800-519-2707).

Shared Family Routine Form

Frequency	Shared routine	Child's input (picks one element or activity)	Parent's input (picks one element or activity)
Daily			
Weekly			
Monthly			
Yearly			

Your parent is working on improving communication skills with you. This week we have asked your parent to make time to talk with you about your day at school. This may be something you and your parent already do, or it may be new. Either way, when your parent has talked with you, fill out the rating sheet below about how well your mom or dad did.

What did you talk about?

_____

_____

_____

_____

Was it easy to talk with your parent?

☐ Yes   ☐ No

Did your parent . . .

show understanding?	☐ Yes	☐ No
summarize what you said?	☐ Yes	☐ No
show patience?	☐ Yes	☐ No
act positive?	☐ Yes	☐ No

Do you think your parent listened to you?

☐ Yes   ☐ No

What could your parent do to make communication better between the two of you?

_____

_____

_____

_____

_____

Child's signature

For: _____ Child's Age: _____ Date: _____

Youth Adjustment

Behavior

Emotional Adjustment

Peer Relationships

School Success

Coping and Self-Management

Other (describe): _____

10	9	8	7	6	5	4	3	2	1
Strength							Needs Attention		

Family Background and Support

Family Stress

Parent Well-Being

Parent Coping Strategies

Caring Adults/Support Network

Partner Support

Parent Substance Use

Other (describe): _____

10	9	8	7	6	5	4	3	2	1
Strength							Needs Attention		

Family Management and Relationships

Relationship Quality

Positive Parenting

Monitoring

Limit Setting

Problem Solving/Communication

Other (describe): _____

10	9	8	7	6	5	4	3	2	1
Strength							Needs Attention		

References

Barlow, D.H. (2004). Psychological treatments. *American Psychologist, 59*(9), 869–878.

Bijou, S.W. (1993). *Behavior analysis of child development* (2nd rev.). Reno, NV: Context Press.

Chamberlain, P., & Moore, K.J. (1998). Models of community treatment for serious offenders. In J. Crane (Ed.), *Social programs that work* (pp. 258–276). Princeton, NJ: Russell Sage.

Conger, R.D., Wallace, L.E., Sun, Y., Simons, R.L., McLoyd, V.C., & Brody, G.H. (2002). Economic pressure in African American families: A replication and extension of the family stress model. *Developmental Psychology, 38*, 179–192.

Dishion, T.J., & Andrews, D.W. (1995). Preventing escalation in problem behaviors with high-risk young adolescents: Immediate and 1-year outcomes. *Journal of Consulting and Clinical Psychology, 63*, 538–548.

Dishion, T.J., Andrews, D.W., Kavanagh, K., & Soberman, L.H. (1996). Preventive interventions for high-risk youth: The Adolescent Transitions Program. In R.D. Peters & R.J. McMahon (Eds.), *Preventing childhood disorders, substance abuse, and delinquency* (pp. 184–214). Thousand Oaks, CA: Sage.

Dishion, T.J., & Kavanagh, K. (2003). *Intervening in adolescent problem behavior: A family-centered approach.* New York: Guilford.

Dishion, T.J., Kavanagh, K., & Dionne, R. (1998, November). *The Family Check-Up: A brief intervention for families with young adolescents.* Workshop presented at the 32nd annual convention of the Association for Advancement of Behavior Therapy, Washington, DC.

Dishion, T.J., Knutson, N.M., Brauer, L., Gill, A., Risso, J., & Kavanagh, K. (2010). *The COACH system for observing and supporting fidelity and effectiveness in the implementation of the EcoFIT model.* Unpublished manuscript available from Child and Family Center, 195 W. 12th Ave., Eugene, OR 97401.

Dishion, T.J., McCord, J., & Poulin, F. (1999). When interventions harm: Peer groups and problem behavior. *American Psychologist, 54*, 755–764.

Dishion, T.J., & McMahon, R.J. (1999). Parental monitoring and the prevention of problem behavior: A conceptual and empirical reformulation. In R.S. Ashery (Ed.), *Research meeting on drug abuse prevention through family interventions* (NIDA

Research Monograph No. 177, pp. 229–259). Washington, DC: U.S. Government Printing Office.

Dishion, T.J., & Patterson, G.R. (1999). Model-building in developmental psychopathology: A pragmatic approach to understanding and intervention. *Journal of Clinical Child Psychology, 28*, 502–512.

Dishion, T.J., Reid, J.B., & Patterson, G.R. (1988). Empirical guidelines for a family intervention for adolescent drug use. In R.E. Coombs (Ed.), *The family context of adolescent drug use* (pp. 189–224). New York: Haworth.

Dishion, T.J., Shaw, D.S., Connell, A.M., Gardner, F., Weaver, C.M., & Wilson, M.N. (2008). The Family Check-Up with high-risk indigent families: Preventing problem behavior by increasing parents' positive behavior support in early childhood. *Child Development, 79*(5), 1395–1414.

Dishion, T.J., & Stormshak, E. (2007). *Intervening in children's lives: An ecological, family-centered approach to mental health care.* Washington, DC: American Psychological Association.

Eddy, J.M., Reid, J.B., Stoolmiller, M., & Fetrow, R.A. (2003). Outcomes during middle school for an elementary school–based preventive intervention for conduct problems: Follow-up results from a randomized trial. *Behavior Therapy, 34*, 535–552.

Elder, G.H., Caspi, A., & Van Nguyen, T. (1986). Resourceful and vulnerable children: Family influences in hard times. In R.K. Silbereisen, K. Eyferth, & G. Rudinger (Eds.), *Development as action in context: Problem behavior and normal youth development* (pp. 167–186). New York: Springer-Verlag.

Forgatch, M.S., Bullock, B.M., & Patterson, G.R. (2004). From theory to practice: Increasing effective parenting through role play. The Oregon Model of Parent Management Training (PMTO). In H. Steiner, K. Chang, J. Lock, & J. Wilson (Eds.), *Handbook of mental health interventions in children and adolescents: An integrated development approach* (pp. 782–813). San Francisco: Jossey-Bass.

Forgatch, M.S., & Patterson, G.R. (2010). Parent management training–Oregon model: An intervention for antisocial behavior in children and adolescents. In J.R. Weisz & A.E. Kazdin (Eds.), *Evidence-based psychotherapies for children and adolescents* (pp. 159–178). New York: Guilford Press.

Forgatch, M.S., Patterson, G.R., & DeGarmo, D.S. (2005). Evaluating fidelity: Predictive validity for a measure of competent adherence to the Oregon Model of Parent Management Training. *Behavior Therapy, 36*, 3–13.

Forgatch, M.S., Patterson, G.R., & Skinner, M.L. (1988). A mediational model for the effect of divorce on antisocial behavior in boys. In E.M. Hetherington & J.D. Aresteh (Eds.), *Impact of divorce, single parenting, and step-parenting on children* (pp. 135–154). Hillsdale, NJ: Erlbaum.

Hayes, S.C., Strosahl, K.D., & Wilson, K.G. (1999). *Acceptance and commitment therapy: An experimental approach to behavior change.* New York: Guilford.

Henggeler, S.W., & Lee, T. (2003). Multisystemic treatment of serious clinical problems. In A.E. Kazdin & J.R. Weisz (Eds.), *Evidence-based psychotherapies for adolescents* (pp. 301–322). New York: Guilford.

Henggeler, S.W., & Schaeffer, C. (2010). Treating serious antisocial behavior using multisystemic therapy. In J.R. Weisz & A.E. Kazdin (Eds.), *Evidence-based psychotherapies for children and adolescents* (pp. 259–276). New York: Guilford.

Henggeler, S., Schoenwald, S., Borduin, C., Rowland, M., & Cunningham, P. (1998). *Multisystemic treatment of antisocial behavior in children and adolescents.* New York: Guilford.

Hetherington, E.M. (1988). Coping with family transitions: Winners, losers and survivors. *Child Development, 60,* 1–14.

Kazdin, A.E. (1995). Bridging child, adolescent, and adult psychotherapy: Directions for research. *Psychotherapy Research, 5*(3), 258–277.

Kazdin, A.E. (2010). Problem-solving skills training and parent management training for oppositional defiant disorder and conduct disorder. In J.R. Weisz & A.E. Kazdin (Eds.), *Evidence-based psychotherapies for children and adolescents* (pp. 211–226). New York: Guilford Press.

Kellam, S.G. (1990). Developmental epidemiological framework for family research on depression and aggression. In G.R. Patterson (Ed.), *Depression and aggression in family interaction: Advances in family research* (pp. 11–48). Hillsdale, NJ: Erlbaum.

Kaminski, J.W., Valle, L.A., Filene, J.H., & Boyle, C.L. (2008). A meta-analytic review of components associated with parent training program effectiveness. *Journal of Abnormal Child Psychology, 36,* 567–589.

Liddle, H.A. (2010). Treating adolescent substance abuse using multidimensional family therapy. In J.R. Weisz & A.E. Kazdin (Eds.), *Evidence-based psychotherapies for children and adolescents* (pp. 416–432). New York: Guilford Press.

Linehan, M.M. (2000). The empirical basis of dialectical behavior therapy: Development of new treatments versus evaluation of existing treatments. *Clinical Psychology: Science and Practice, 7*(1), 113–119.

Miller, W.R., & Rollnick, S. (2002). *Motivational interviewing: Preparing people for change* (2nd ed.). New York: Guilford.

Patterson, G.R. (1973). Changes in status of family members as controlling stimuli: A basis for describing treatment process. In L.A. Hamerlynck, L.C. Handy, & E.J. Mash (Eds.), *Behavior change: Methodology, concepts, and practices* (pp. 169–191). Champaign, IL: Research Press.

Patterson, G.R. (1974). Interventions for boys with conduct problems: Multiple settings, treatments, and criteria. *Journal of Consulting and Clinical Psychology 42,* 471–481.

Patterson, G.R. (1982). *A social learning approach: III. Coercive family process.* Eugene, OR: Castalia.

Patterson, G.R., & Forgatch, M.S. (1985). Therapist behavior as a determinant for client resistance: A paradox for the behavior modifier. *Journal of Consulting and Clinical Psychology, 53*(6), 846–851.

Patterson, G.R., & Reid, J.B. (1984). Social interactional processes within the family: The study of moment-by-moment family transactions in which human development is embedded. *Journal of Applied Developmental Psychology, 5,* 237–262.

Patterson, G.R., Reid, J.B., & Dishion, T.J. (1992). *Antisocial boys.* Eugene, OR: Castalia.

Patterson, G., Reid, J., Jones, R., & Conger, R. (1975). *A social learning approach to family intervention: Families with aggressive children.* Eugene, OR: Castalia.

Reid, J.B. (1978). *A social learning approach to family intervention: Observation in home settings* (Vol. 2). Eugene, OR: Castalia.

Shaw, D.S., Dishion, T.J., Supplee, L., Gardner, F., & Arnds, K. (2006). Randomized trial of a family-centered approach to the prevention of early conduct problems: Two-year effects of the Family Check-Up in early childhood. *Journal of Consulting and Clinical Psychology, 74*(1), 1–9.

Shaw, D.S., Gilliom, M., Ingoldsby, E.M., & Nagin, D. (2003). Trajectories leading to school-age conduct problems. *Developmental Psychology, 39*, 189–200.

Smith, D.K., & Chamberlain, P. (2010). Multidimensional treatment foster care for adolescents: Processes and outcomes. In J.R. Weisz & A.E. Kazdin (Eds.), *Evidence-based psychotherapies for children and adolescents* (pp. 243–258). New York: Guilford Press.

Snyder, J., Reid, J.B., & Patterson, G.R. (2003). A social learning model of child and adolescent antisocial behavior. In B.B. Lahey, T.E. Moffitt, & A. Caspi (Eds.), *Causes of conduct disorder and juvenile delinquency* (pp. 27–48). New York: Guilford Press.

Stormshak, E.A., & Dishion, T.J. (2002). An ecological approach to child and family clinical and counseling psychology. *Clinical Child and Family Psychology Review, 5*(3), 197–215.

Waldron, H.B., & Brody, J.L. (2010). Functional family therapy for adolescent substance use disorders. In J.R. Weisz & A.E. Kazdin (Eds.), *Evidence-based psychotherapies for children and adolescents* (pp. 401–415). New York: Guilford Press.

Webster-Stratton, C., & Reid, M.J. (2010). The Incredible Years Parents, Teachers, and Children Training Series: A multifaceted treatment approach for young children with conduct disorders. In J.R. Weisz & A.E. Kazdin (Eds.), *Evidence-based psychotherapies for children and adolescents* (pp. 194–210). New York: Guilford Press.

Zisser, A., & Eyberg, S.M. (2010). Parent–child interaction therapy and the treatment of disruptive behavior disorders. In J.R. Weisz & A.E. Kazdin (Eds.), *Evidence-based psychotherapies for children and adolescents* (pp. 179–193). New York: Guilford Press.

About the Authors

THOMAS J. DISHION is a professor of psychology at Arizona State University and a research scientist at the Child and Family Center at the University of Oregon. His research focuses on the role of parenting in the development of adjustment problems in children, as well as on the development of interventions for families and children, such as the Family Check-Up. He has spearheaded several randomized studies evaluating the effects of family-centered interventions over the past 25 years. He has published more than 160 scientific reports on these topics, a book for parents on family management, and three books for professionals working with troubled children and their families.

ELIZABETH A. STORMSHAK is a professor in counseling psychology in the College of Education at the University of Oregon and director of the Child and Family Center. Her primary research focus is on the prevention of problem behavior in early and middle childhood, including substance abuse, conduct problems, and academic failure. She has received multiple federal grants to develop and implement prevention programs for early and middle childhood. Her research focuses on refining clinical models to engage families in the intervention process and enhance long-term, positive outcomes for youth.

KATHRYN A. KAVANAGH is at the Child and Family Center at the University of Oregon. For the past 30 years, she has been engaged in the study of family processes related to healthy outcomes for children and adolescents and in developing effective intervention programs from those findings. Currently, her primary research focus is the translation of evidence-based practices to community settings such as public schools, workplaces, and community mental health agencies. She has received funding to develop several media-based intervention programs for children and families and has published books and scientific articles on these topics.